a more **mystical** approach to pain management

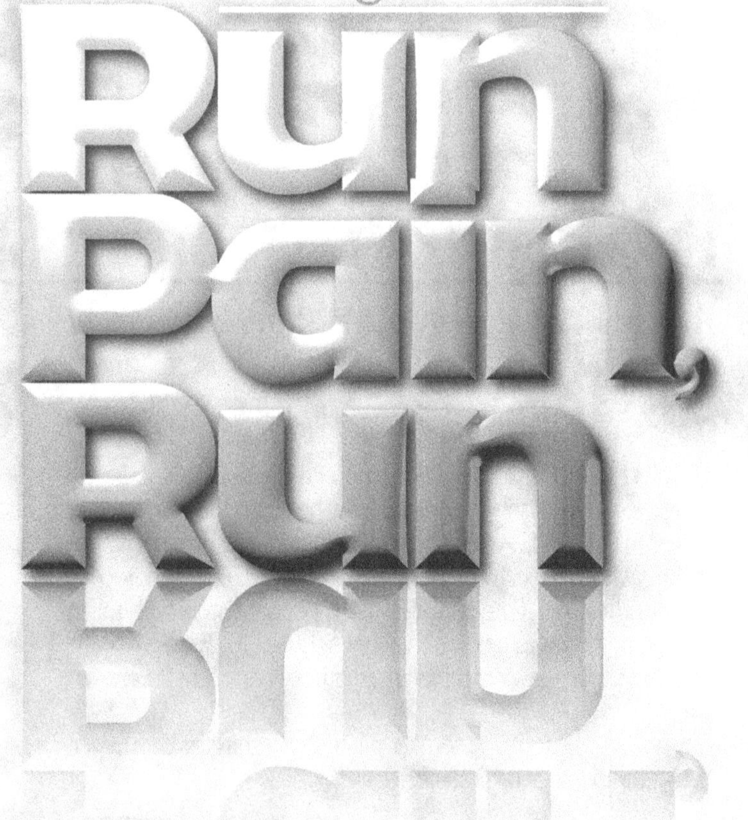

Thirtysix.org & Shaarnum Productions

Run Pain, Run

A More Mystical Approach to Pain Management

ISBN 9798346632184

Any questions should be sent to: pinchasw@thirtysix.org. Cover background image by Freepik.

Published by:
Thirtysix.org & Shaarnun Productions
22 Yitzchak Road
Telzstone, Kiryat Yearim
Israel   9083800

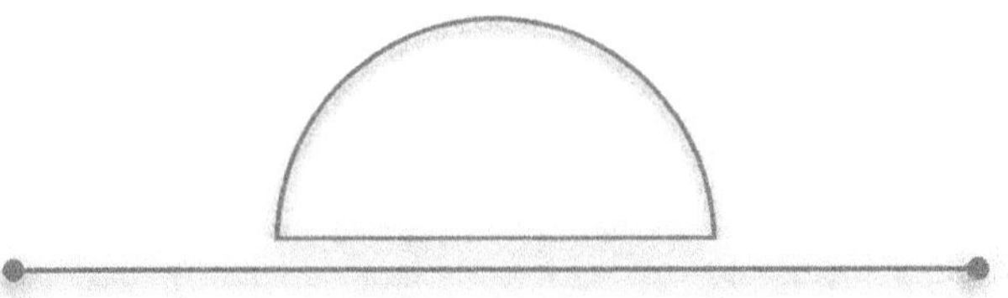

Dedicated in memory of
the holy Rav Gedalia Moshe
son of the holy Rav Shlomo, z"l
of Zvil.

The Beliak Family

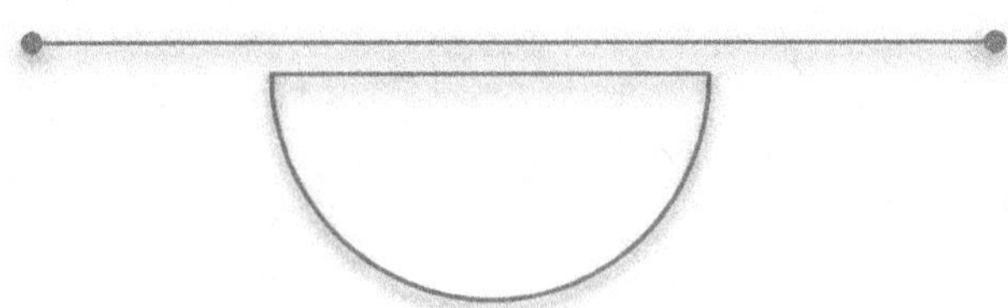

Contents

intro

e were not born into pain. It was a consequence of the sin of eating from the *Aitz HaDa'as Tov v'Ra*. That led to expulsion from Paradise into a world of pain and suffering. We're obviously able to enjoy ourselves a lot in this world, but compared to the pleasure of *Gan Aiden*, what we're lacking is also part of the pain of this world.

It's a great motivator, pain is. It's just that it doesn't always motivate us in the right spiritual direction. Usually it doesn't. We believe that we shouldn't have to suffer and resent it when we do. Therefore, we are devoted to avoiding pain and feel justified in being so. Even if we accept that pain is an unavoidable part of life, most people don't accept that it is a necessary part of life.

This means that even though we have motivational

statements like *"no pain, no gain,"* people spend so much time and energy trying to gain without pain. And even though we are told, *"According to the suffering is the reward"* (*Pirkei Avos* 5:23), we look for ways to get reward without suffering.

It's a body thing. The pain we fear most is the kind felt by the body. The body was not built for comfort, but it certainly became that way after leaving the comfort of Paradise. Once, we had skin like light—*kasnos ohr*[1]—and our bodies were more like souls. But then we sinned and were transformed, resulting in bodies made from skin—*kasnos ohr*.[2]

That's when pain became a thing for us. For her share in the sin, God told Chava:

> *I will increase your sorrow and your pregnancy; in pain you shall bear children.* (*Bereishis* 3:16)

Before the sin, childbirth was easy, quick, and pleasant. Not so after. Before the sin, food was also an entirely different experience. After the sin, this applied:

> *By the sweat of your brow, you will eat bread...* (*Bereishis* 3:19)

---

[1] *Aleph-Vav-Raish*, which means *light*.
[2] *Ayin-Vav-Raish*, which means *skin*.

And though we can now buy bread without sweating much, we still have to "sweat" to make the money to pay for it. Regardless, the bottom line is that the world outside of *Gan Aiden* is one in which we must expend energy and time, having lost immortality as well, and both of which we have limited quantities.

The rest of history since has been about beating the rap. It has been about finding the perfect painkillers in whatever form they may come. To live is to know pain, but to know painkillers is to lessen that pain, perhaps even manage it, to try and maintain some level of pleasure nevertheless.

Because we were made for pleasure. We were created in Paradise, and it is to Paradise that we long to return. Desperate to get back, we grasp at whatever aspect of Paradise we can find…often at great sacrifice to life itself, in this world, and, more importantly, in the next world, the real gain of our pain in the here and now.

It turns out that the difference between a great person and an average one is the pain they are prepared to live with to accomplish meaningful goals. A great person may fear pain like the next person, but they also know better than to just run away from it. They may not embrace pain (who does?), but they try hard not to let it get in the way of doing ultimately meaningful things.

Even more so, they understand and appreciate that the pain is not a sideshow but part of the main event. We were sent packing from *Gan Aiden* for *tikun*, our rectification, and the world's rectification. If we left with pain, it was because we needed to accomplish both.

One year, I herniated a disk in my back. It had been happening for years, but it only took two days to become the most excruciating pain I have ever known—even on prescription painkillers they keep in a safe. You don't know how well-protected nerves are in the body until they no longer are.

Not only was the pain terrible and demoralizing but there was no position I could take that eased it even a little. Something as simple as getting off the sofa and walking a couple of feet to the bathroom was torture. Basic daily activities become almost impossible tasks.

It was the first time I could see why some people with incurable pain would choose to end their lives instead. I could see why someone not concerned about a Torah prohibition against suicide would choose death over such debilitating pain, especially if they believed it would never go away. What kind of life is it when death seems more appealing?

I am obviously not the first person to ask that question, and certainly not the last. And whatever pain I suffered over the six weeks to recovery, I did recover, *thank God*. As traumatic as my pain was, it was not traumatic enough to remain an active memory past a year. So many others have it far worse.

But everything in life is relative. Sadness is sadness, even if the reason for one person's seems so much more trivial than the reason for another's. Suffering is suffering, even if one person's suffering seems so minimal compared to the suffering of another. Externals vary from person to person and from moment to moment. But each of us lives life based upon our perception of it, and that is personal and in the brain.

The difference is in the outcome. Someone can believe that their world is coming to an end because of something but quickly finds out otherwise simply because they exaggerated their problem. For others, the problem may end up being as serious as they thought and actually beyond recovery as they feared.

But for the period that both their brains perceived an insurmountable problem, they were equally distressed. They were both faced with the same decision, and that was what to do about life with the problem. They had to decide what to do about their pain…how to live with it and despite it.

The question is as old as man himself. It's the answer that keeps changing from generation to generation.

one

So many decisions are made today out of pain, or to avoid it. People have always done that, some more than others. But there have been times when many have been willing to bite the bullet to do the right thing, especially when it came to the larger issues in history.

For a long time, the Arabs did not care about world opinion. They only cared about what they wanted—the State of Israel, and had no problem causing problems for others to get it. They had their allies and military support, and tried everything they could to beat the Jewish State through war.

But it didn't work, *thank God*. There were close calls, but in the end, Israel survived Arab attacks who were no further ahead than when they started, except for the death and damage they caused. Their military strategy proved to be ineffective, and they became extremely frustrated.

I don't know exactly when, but they figured out that they could get the world to do to Israel through political pressure what they could not do to through military operations. I don't know who told them, but they realized that they could wear down the rest of the world quicker and more easily than they can Israel, and that could force Israel to make concessions.

That's what the Arabs did, and that is what they're doing. They're making their problem the world's problem, so that nations will take up the Palestinian's cause just to end the negative and taxing impact the Middle East is having on their peace of mind. Right or wrong, the world will do whatever it must to restore balance as quickly as possible, and they'll choose the path of least resistance.

The Arabs have never been easy to appease. They have never been a compromising people, especially since Islam became their official religion. You either give them, what they want or pay the price for saying no, and 9/11 was a tragic example of that.

Israel, on the other hand, is a tiny nation. Secular Israelis yearn to be part of the family of nations as an equal and hate it when they're rejected. Whereas Arabs sell very little to get what they want, secular Jews will and do sell their souls to fulfill their personal and international ambitions. They are, by default, the path of least resistance, and if not for *Hashgochah Pratis* (Divine Providence) they would have capitulated to world demands everywhere they could.

For so many reasons, some historic and some moral, the Arabs don't have a case. They have already been indulged more than they should have, but it has made no difference. Any logical well-balanced person who took the time to learn the details of the struggle and check out the facts on the ground, would support the Israelis. Some already have, and some already do.

But the world does not work that way today. Once, if you want to know the truth, you had to go looking for it. Today, people are fed information, and often by unreliable sources. Privilege has made people lazy and made them desperate for meaning. Falsehood is rampant, truth is personal, and intellectual vulnerability is great. The Palestinians couldn't have found a better time or marketplace for their brand of reality.

Should we be surprised? Really? In a world that spends so much money on food, clothing, and entertainment? In a world that places such an emphasis on physical appearance over personality traits? Somewhere the *Sitra Achra* sits in a penthouse office at the top of some skyscraper, feet up on the desk relishing how far mankind has unwittingly gone down his path.

It's a *yetzer hara's* world out there. That says it all. So much of what goes on from day to day is just to cater to the instinctual drives of people. Few people look at this world as the corridor to the World to Come that it is supposed to be,[1] but as the World to Come itself, which is true for many but it is not supposed to be true for the Jewish people.[2]

But the difference between a Jew and a non-Jew becomes nominal once a Jew stops believing in Torah from Sinai, or God Himself. They will tell you themselves that they want it to be that way, and would much rather invest in a comfortable life in this world than save up for one they can't believe exists. So they too end up choosing the path of least resistance, prepared to sell the soul of their land and people to get the world off their back.

If people don't believe in God, can they be expected to act otherwise? If people doubt there is a higher cause, can they be expected to sacrifice for one? If this is all there is, and so many people suspect it is, why suffer without gain? Work hard for money to have fun? Sure. Work out in the gym harder to increase your chances of victory on the field, why not?

People will even make the tough choice for a "moral" value they personally relate to, like go to *shul* on *Yom Kippur* because that it is what their family always did. They'll begrudgingly do the "right" thing if all of society says to if only not to rock the boat.

But painfully do the right thing as defined by some invisible being for reward in some hitherto unproven future paradise? Isn't that the very *definition* of delusional? It

---

[1] *Pirkei Avos* 4:16.
[2] *Avodah Zarah* 10b.

is according to all the people who look at those who do as, well, delusional, and they want nothing to do with them.

The strange thing is that, for the most part, the feeling is mutual. The Orthodox world prefers to be left alone to do its own thing, leaving others to do theirs. They see the lifestyle of their non-religious brothers and criticize it among themselves. But aside from a few zealots here and there, they do not confront them about it.

Yet confrontation there is. A lot of it. It's even vicious at times. It's as if an invisible gravitational force draws them together while they fight to be apart from one another. The dislike of one another is obvious, so it doesn't make people wonder about the situation…until they realize it shouldn't be as obvious as it is.

This story explains the pain. There is the story of Amnon and Tamar in *Tanach*, a son and daughter of Dovid *HaMelech* from different mothers.[3] It is reported that Amnon became so obsessed with his step-sister that he feigned illness to be alone with her in order to be intimate, which he was.

But rather than love and marry her as she begged him to do now that she had been disgraced, Amnon rejected Tamar. And not only did Amnon no longer *love* Tamar, but it says that his hatred for her was greater than any love he had for her, quite the reversal.

The truth is, Amnon had only been infatuated with

---

[3] I *Shmuel* 13:1.

Tamar, which is why he quickly disliked her once he had fulfilled his selfish desire. But his hatred for Tamar? She had done nothing that was hateful! But he had, and every time he saw Tamar he was reminded of his own loathsome act, and that made him feel bad about himself.

And hate her. Since Tamar's very existence made Amnon feel bad about himself, he had to make a choice. Either he had to do *teshuvah* and somehow compensate Tamar for what he had put her through, or he had to get rid of her. As to be expected, he cowardly chose to get rid of Tamar.

This also explains why it is not enough for many secular Jews to just leave it as "to each his own." Orthodox Jews do not have to actually publicly say something to criticize secular Jews. For many, their very presence and existence is enough to do that, causing some non-religious Jews to feel bad about themselves.

On the rarest of occasions, that has caused some secular Jews to reconsider their way of life and return over time to a more Torah lifestyle. Others, either because they are not conscious of why they feel as they do, or don't want to be, blame their feelings of guilt on their perceived cause of it. Taking the path of least resistance, they turn against religious Jews and not themselves.

Because, though you can take the Jew out of Judaism, can you really take the Judaism out of a Jew? Maybe for some. We do have a concept of *kares*, of being cut off from the Jewish people. It's a Torah punishment, but more of a consequence of separating body and soul so much that, for all intents and purposes, the spiritual tether keeping them together goes snap.

Completely? Permanently?

There are varying opinions about that, as well as how responsible a person has to be for their sin before it might actually happen. It is a very confusing and confused world, and some people who might have once seemed completely cut off from Judaism have actually come back, against all the odds.

Others have not been so fortunate. Judaism was grossly misrepresented in their early years, and growing with faulty assumptions have led to distorted perceptions. If Divine Providence doesn't arrange for them to see this and change those assumptions, then they live and die with those perceptions—and out of touch with their inner Jewish self.

Consequently, they can easily mistake that inner sense of disgust as being the result of those who live Jewishly, when it is really because of those who do not. But while that may explain the situation to us, it is rare when a secular Jew investigates and realizes this, and then moves in the other direction.

One such rare individual was once considered to be the "Johnny Carson" of Israel. Uri Zohar had his own talk show, made movies, and had many, many devoted admirers. He had also been super secular and quite anti-Charedi. He was the quintessential modern Israeli Jew, worldly and with the times.

His autobiography tells the story of his remarkable and miraculous transition from his world to our world, and it certainly didn't happen overnight. But when it did, the shock waves it sent through the secular Israeli world classified as a major quake, a ten on the psychological and emotional Richter Scale.

Uri Zohar was a quick study and rose up in the ranks of outreach, devoting himself to trying to save as many fellow Israelis from making the same mistake he almost made. His level of success was amazing, and its effects will be felt for generations to come.

Uri Zohar, *zt"l*, died a legend, though not the kind he started out as. And his story is somewhat reminiscent of another one in the *Gemora*, this one about one Rabbi Shimon *ben* Lakish, otherwise known as Reish Lakish:

One day, Rebi Yochanan was bathing in the Jordan [River]. Reish Lakish saw him and jumped into the Jordan, pursuing him. [Rebi Yochanan] said [to Reish Lakish]: "Your strength [is fit] for Torah!"

[Reish Lakish] said to him: "Your beauty [is fit] for women!"

[Rabbi Yochanan] said to him: If you return [to the pursuit of Torah], I will give you my sister [in marriage], who is more beautiful than I am!"

[Reish Lakish] accepted. (*Bava Metzia* 84a)

It is hard to imagine how someone like Reish Lakish could start out on a Torah path so late in life and rise to become the great Rebi Yochanan's *chavrusa*, but he did. So did the great Rebi Akiva as well, who once told his *talmidim*:

> When I was a simpleton I said, "Who will give me a *talmid chacham* so that I can bite him like a donkey?" (*Pesachim* 49b)

Such animosity! But from what, if Rebi Akiva *already* kept all the *mitzvos*?

Because a *talmid chacham* was a reminder to Akiva *ben* Yosef that he could be more, *should* be more, that he could one day be the great Rebi Akiva. Not yet being in a position to be, it *hurt* and that, over time, turns into resentment.

But Akiva *ben* Yosef did not take the path of least resistance and stay hateful, and that's why he eventually became the great Rebi Akiva. Shimon ben Lakish accepted his need to be better, and merited to be the *chavrusa* of the *Gadol HaDor*, Rebi Yochanan.

And people like Uri Zohar over the ages who have been brave enough to confront their spiritual lackings have merited to turn their enemies into their allies. They were strong enough to return to the spiritual drawing board and start again, the correct and eternal way. What a *zechus*!

It will happen to the rest of mankind once the final

War of Gog and Magog takes place. That is the entire reason for it, to fulfill the verse of *"On that day, God will be One and His Name, One."*[4] Thousands of years of faulty assumptions that have led to faulty perceptions will crumble before the clearest of truths. Who will survive the transition depends upon who will have the strength at that time to accept the change.

---

[4] *Zechariah* 14:9.

two

There are so many things about the way this world works that beg the question, *why?* The answer, according to *Hashkofah* 101 to 404, is always because it is the best kind of world to support the creation of man and free will.

Why is it the best world for all of that? The answer this time is, *we don't know*. We really don't. As much as we do know and as sophisticated as our knowledge may be, we can't answer that question unless God does first.

Because if God had created us already in the World to Come with only a memory of having lived in this world as if we did, would we know the difference? Would we care if we did? Wouldn't it be like going on vacation without having to work first?

And if you ask, "But would we enjoy it as much?" the

answer is, we *could*. Because, just as we were made to enjoy reward more after working for it, God could have made us able to enjoy reward *without* working for it, and we would. He just chose not to…for our sake.

Because God is the *Ultimate* Good,[1] and only does the *ultimate* good. So if God made the world this way, with all of its rules and circumstances it is not only good, but *ultimately* good…no matter how flawed Creation seems to us and history demands revision.

The *Gemora* speaks about *yesurim*—suffering—a fair bit, like here for example:

Rebi Eliezer fell ill, and his students came to visit him. [Rebi Eliezer] told them: "There is intense anger in the world, [and it is because of the anger of The Holy One, Blessed is He, that I am suffering. His students] began to cry [because of his suffering], but Rebi Akiva laughed. So they asked him: "Why are you laughing?"

[Rebi Akiva] asked [back]: "Why do you cry?"

They answered: "Is it possible that [Rebi Eliezer], a [virtual] Torah scroll is in pain and we will not cry?"

Rebi Akiva told them: "This is why I laugh, because as long as I saw that. for my teacher. his wine does not ferment and spoil, his flax is not stricken, his oil does not spoil, and his honey does not turn rancid, I thought that, *God forbid*, my teacher has already re-

---

[1] Derech Hashem.

ceived his reward in this world. Now that I see my teacher suffering I can be happy, [because it means that he is receiving punishment in this world for the few sins he may have committed, ensuring that he will receive a complete reward in the World-to-Come]!" (*Sanhedrin* 101a)

From this we learn how suffering is a way to pay dues in this world in order to receive reward in the next world. The *Gemora* says it here specifically:

To what are the righteous in this world compared? To a tree that is standing entirely in a pure place and its branches hang over an impure place. If its branches are cut, it will stand entirely in a pure place. So too, The Holy One, Blessed is He, brings suffering upon the righteous in this world [to cleanse them of their few sins. He makes them suffer] so that they will inherit the World-to-Come. (*Kiddushin* 40b)

And because He likes to hear from us:

The Holy One, Blessed is He desired to hear their voices, but they were unwilling. What did The Holy One, Blessed is He do? He hardened Pharaoh's heart and he pursued them. This is what it says: *"God hardened the heart of Pharaoh king of Egypt, and he pursued"* (*Shemos* 14:8), and it says: *"Pharaoh ap-*

proached" (*Shemos* 14:10). What is "approached— *hikriv"*? He brought the Jewish people closer—*hikriv* —to *teshuvah*. When they saw [Pharaoh and his army], they looked to The Holy One, Blessed is He, and they cried out before Him, as it says: *"The Children of Israel raised their eyes and, behold, the Egyptians were traveling after them and they were very frightened; the Children of Israel cried out to God"* (*Shemos* 14:10) with the same cry that they cried out in Egypt. Once The Holy One, Blessed is He heard, He said: *"Had I not done this to you, I would not have heard your voice."* Regarding this moment, He said: *"My dove, in the clefts of the rock…let Me your voice"* (*Shir HaShirim* 2:14). It does not say, "let me hear a voice," but "your voice," the voice that I heard in Egypt. When the Children of Israel cried out before The Holy One, Blessed is He, immediately, *"God saved [the Jewish people] on that day"* (*Shemos* 14:30). (*Shir HaShirim Rabbah* 2:6)

Well that makes sense, sort of. God loves to hear from us, but we forget to talk to Him…until He reminds us Who runs the world, and how much we depend upon Him for peace of mind. Then, hurting, we talk to God once again, He is happy to hear from us, and there is "peace on all of Israel."

But couldn't He just call us, without sending us pain?

Apparently not, or He would. Somehow pain is such

an integral part of Creation and history that God built it in. Most people think that pain was just an unforeseeable and unnecessary consequence of Adam *HaRishon's* tragic mistake. Yes, God created it or it wouldn't exist, but planned for?

Yes, *planned* for, from the *beginning*. Man is imperfect and man makes mistakes, but God is not and does not. Pain was not some contingency plan in case man didn't get it right. It was all planned and staged out, including man not getting it right:

> *"Go and see the works of God, awesome in deed toward mankind."* (*Tehillim* 66:5): Go and see how when The Holy One, Blessed is He, created the world, He created the Angel of Death on the *first* day…Man, however, was created on the *sixth* day, and yet death was blamed on him. To what is this similar? To a man who wants to divorce his wife and writes her a *Get*, after which he returns home holding the *Get*, looking for a pretext[2] to give it to her. He tells her, *"Prepare me a drink."*
>
> She does, and taking it from her he says, *"Here is your Get."*
>
> She asks, *"What is this?"*
>
> He then tells her, *"Leave my house since you made me a warm drink,"* to which she replies, *"How did*

---

2 The Hebrew word is "alillah."

you know in advance that I would prepare you a warm drink that you were able to write a Get and come home with it?"

So too Adam said to The Holy One, Blessed is He, "Master of the Universe! The Torah was with You for 2000 years before You even created the world…And yet it instructs, *'This is the law when a man will die in a tent'* (*Bamidbar* 19:14). If You had not *already* decided that death should be in Creation, would You have written this? Rather, You were just looking for a pretext to blame death on me!" This is what is meant by *"awesome in deed."* (*Tanchuma, Vayaishev* 4)

Certainly if death was destined to be part of history, then pain as well. For God, being above time and having no future or past, everything that will ever be has already happened. And all free will issues aside, the question becomes, *what is so primordially good about pain that it had to be an integral part of the equation of life?*

The answer is not short. Just the opposite, it is very complicated and complex, tied to the *kabbalistic* explanation of how God went about making Creation. But if you *really, really* want to understand pain, you have to first understand this.

It is called *Hispashtus* and *Histalkus*, Emanation and Withdrawal. First Divine light emanates and is then pulled back, only to emanate again, and then be pulled back again. This is the way God made the world, and that is the process He has used to add to Creation ever since.[3]

In fact, it seems to be built into life. Very often in life the first time does not succeed but it does lay the foundation for the second time. True, being human, we're bound to make uncalculated mistakes and learn from them for the next time. There is no question that the spies sent by Yehoshua after the forty years in the desert learned some important lessons from the ones Moshe sent at the beginning of the forty years.

But God could have made the world differently. He could have made man more perfect, and there are plenty of times when *Hashgochah Pratis* has made sure that something has succeeded the first time, even against incredible odds. But it is not the general way of the world, to the point that a person can almost expect to fail the first time at anything. *Histalkus* seems as much a part of Creation as *hispashtus*.

So even though there is an angel that teaches all of

---

[3] Before our world existed there was only *Ohr Ain Sof,* God's Infinite Light. As the name implies, it was a uniformly infinite light within which nothing created can exist, the opposite of what God wanted. So He did something we don't understand but completely depend upon, and that is applied the concept of *tzimtzum* and constricted His light by withdrawing it from a certain area, leaving but a *roshem* —impression. Everything beyond this newly created *challal*—hollow—was *Ohr Ain Sof,* and free of any kind of boundary or measurement. Inside the *Challal* however was the opposite reality, *only* measurement and boundary, without which we can neither exist nor make any kind of difference to reality.

Torah while still in the womb—*hispashtus*, he makes us forget it all at birth—*histalkus*.[4] In the end, is anything gained, and if no, then why teach it to us in the first place?

Because each time a light is pulled back, it leaves something behind. We forget the knowledge at birth, but we don't lose it. Rather, it seems to sink into our unconscious mind, making learning the process of taking knowledge from the unconscious mind, and everyone knows that it is much easier to remember old knowledge that learn new knowledge.

Furthermore, we tend to more strongly acquire that which we work for than what we are given for free. And it is precisely that relationship that unifies us with the knowledge so that we don't only *know* something, but become *one* with it. That is when we go from just *living* life to *being* life.

In the meantime, there is suffering. Every child suffers as they learn. Every businessman has to sweat the details on his way to success. Relationships have ups, but they also have downs, and some are so down that they become too difficult to climb out of.

Because, technical definitions of pain aside, *histalkus* is *hester panim*—the hiding of God's face and withdrawal of His light. When God emanates light, there is *brochah*. When He withdraws it, there is suffering on some level. The desert bloomed when God came down over *Har*

---

[4] *Niddah* 30b.

Sinai. It became a deadly desert again once He withdrew. While Moshe was down in the camp, the Jewish people were like angels. When he "withdrew" to Heaven to receive Torah, the golden calf resulted.

True. But the important thing to remember is that, as much as we'd like the blessing to stay and feel punished when it doesn't, *histalkus* only reduces God's light, not remove it completely. It always leaves something behind, a hidden blessing to prepare us for the next emanation of light that is meant to accomplish even more.

This is the deeper meaning of, "All that God does He does for the good."[5] The world calls it "the silver lining in a cloud," but *kabbalistically* it is more like the *mann* that remained after the dew that covered it "withdrew." It wasn't just bread from Heaven. It was the key to the door that leads us there.[6]

So, unless a person is evil and being punished in this world, all pain, no matter how intense, is the result of a withdrawal of Divine light, but in order to leave something

---

[5] *Brochos* 60b.

[6] The *Gemora* (*Yoma* 75a) discusses the mystical aspects of the mann, and the Torah says, *"He afflicted you and let you go hungry, and then fed you with mann, which you did not know, nor did your forefathers know, so that He would make you know that man does not live by bread alone, but rather, by whatever comes forth from the mouth of God does man live"* (*Devarim* 8:3). The main point of the *mann* was to teach the Jewish people that we survive physically through the spiritual world.

good behind. It is usually not the good we were after, or one that is necessarily recognizable at first. But then again, what we want for ourselves and what God wants for us is often different until we learn why His is the better way.

This is what Rebi Akiva alluded to when he explained himself to Rebi Eliezer. Rebi Eliezer had been suffering but seemed unaware of the good it was doing for him.[7] Even great people need outside opinions to help them see what they cannot. As the *Gemora* says, "A prisoner cannot escape from their own prison."[8]

But once Rebi Akiva explained it, Rebi Eliezer was much better equipped to deal with his situation. He saw the good in his bad, and built upon it, just as he did here:

When they arrived at the Temple Mount, they saw a fox that emerged from the site of the Holy of Holies. They cried, but Rebi Akiva laughed. They asked him:

---

[7] Rebi Akiva added another support that "*yesurim* are to be cherished" from the story of of Menashe who only did *teshuvah* and accepted God once he was made to suffer. This was the realization that Menashe was "left with" once God withdrew his success as a corrupt king and left him with a great sense of vulnerability. People notice and value success and see defeat as a complete loss, overlooking the great insight that it often leaves in its wake. In a world in which physical success is so valued, the insight gained by those who are down and vulnerable is downplayed when, as it is clear from Menashe, it can end being far more valuable and eternal than any material success a person can have.

[8] *Brochos* 5b.

"Why are you laughing?"

So Rebi Akiva asked them: "Why are you crying?"

They answered: "Foxes walk in the place regarding it says: *'The non-priest who approaches shall die'* (*Bamidbar* 1:51), and we shouldn't cry?!"

Rebi Akiva told them: "That is why I am laughing. It says, *'I will take faithful witnesses to Me to attest: Uriah HaKohen, and Zechariah ben Yeverechyahu'* (*Yeshayahu* 8:2). What connection is there between Uriah and Zechariah? Uriah [prophesied] during the First Temple, and Zechariah [prophesied] during the Second Temple. Rather, the verse established that [fulfillment of] the prophecy of Zechariah is dependent [on fulfillment] of the prophecy of Uriah. In Uriah it says: *'Therefore, for your sake Tzion will be plowed as a field, [and Jerusalem will become rubble, and the Temple Mount as the high places of a forest'* (*Michah* 3:12), where foxes are found]. In Zechariah it says: *'There shall yet be elderly men and elderly women sitting in the streets of Jerusalem'* (*Zechariah* 8:4). Until the prophecy of Uriah [with regard to the destruction of the city] was fulfilled I was afraid that the prophecy of Zechariah would not be fulfilled. Now that the prophecy of Uriah was fulfilled, it is evident that the prophecy of Zechariah remains valid!"

They responded him, "Akiva, you have comforted us; Akiva, you have comforted us!" (*Makkos* 24b)

Like most people, the other rabbis with Rebi Akiva saw only the *histalkus* and felt the pain it caused. Rebi Akiva, on the other hand, looked at the situation through the eyes of Kabbalah and knew that every *histalkus*, no matter how punishing, leaves something behind with which to build for the future. He found it, shared, and turned the mood around completely.

Mankind has learned over the millennia that adversity builds good things, and many tales have been told to teach this point. But that doesn't mean that everyone embraces their own personal forms of *histalkus*. On the contrary, the same page of *Gemora* that discusses the good of *yesurim* ends with stories of suffering great rabbis who chose to get out of theirs saying, "I want neither the suffering nor the reward!"

Nevertheless, there is still something else to discuss here, and it is a game changer.

three

The very first test mankind ever went through involved *Da'as*. The very last test mankind will ever go through will involve *Da'as*. And every test mankind will have *ever* gone through between these two points will also have involved *Da'as*, one way or another.

After all, the first test man was put through did not have to do with just *any* tree. It was a tree of *Da'as*, which means that the test was not merely about eating, but about the "eating" of *Da'as*.

That may sound strange at first, but not after this:

The incident with the *Aitz HaDa'as*, regarding which The Holy One, Blessed is He, warned Adam *HaRishon*, involved three [prohibitions]. The first was the actual eating…The second prohibited intimacy, that he should not be intimate with Chava while she was not pure from the latching on of the *Chitzonim*[1]… Intimacy is also referred to as eating, as *Chazal* elucidate in *Bereishis Rabbah* at the end of Ch. 86, on the verse, *"Only the bread which he eats"* (*Bereishis* 39:6)[2] The *mitzvah* was to not be intimate before *Shabbos*, because she was not yet pure from the *Chitzonim*[3]…The third aspect is enlightenment and knowledge, which are included in the language of eating, as in *Yechezkel*: *"Eat this scroll…And He fed me that scroll…Feed your stomach and fill your innards with this scroll…So I ate, and it was as sweet as honey in my mouth"* (*Yechezkel* 3:1-3), and similarly in *Yeshayahu*: *"Go, buy, and eat; go and buy wine and milk without money and without price"* (*Yeshayahu* 55:1). Likewise *Chazal*, in *Shir HaShirim*

---

[1] When man was first created, he was completely pure. Interaction with the snake spiritually defiled them, making procreation problematic since any child conceived would be born with inherent impurity, as was the case with Kayin and Hevel. This was the source of their internal *yetzer hara*, and the reason why expulsion from *Gan Aiden* became imperative. The only way to remove an internal *yetzer hara* is through death, and death was not possible in *Gan Aiden*.

[2] When Yosef rejected the wife of Potiphar he referred to her as the bread her husband eats, a metaphor for intimacy.

[3] *Shabbos* itself would have acted as a means to purify them from the effect of the snake, at which time intimacy would have been a *mitzvah,* and Kayin and Hevel would have been born pure as well.

Rabbah, Ch. 1 compare words of Torah to water, wine, oil, and honey. Thus, enlightenment and knowledge are included in the language of eating, and He [also] warned him not to contemplate or glance at anything to which evil is attached,[4] in order to not be drawn to look into the power of the *Chitzonim* themselves. (*Drushei Olam HaTohu, Drush Aitz HaDa'as, Siman* 3)

The truth is, we do it too. We say things like, "let me digest that information," or "let me mull that over." And just like our digestive system takes in food, separates the good from the bad, and then uses the good while dispensing with the bad, so do our brains. We analyze (digest) what we learn so that we can distinguish the good from the evil, hopefully to use the former and distance ourselves from the latter.

That is what someone made in the image of *Elohim* does:

God said, "Let us make man in our image, after our likeness…And God created man in His image; b'tzelem Elohim—in the image of God He created him…" (Bereishis 1:26)

The term *Elohim* can be used to describe every intel-

---

[4] Such as the *Aitz HaDa'as Tov v'Ra.*

ligent force that is separated from matter…As such, it is eternal, and thus the term is used regarding God and His angels. It is also applied to judges because of their ability to reason. (*Sforno, Bereishis* 1:26)

Because this is the way we get to God in this world. God is Ultimate Truth, but Ultimate Truth is covered by multiple layers that make it imperceptible by many. Even the brightest light becomes invisible when closed off to the world.

But when a person goes in pursuit of truth, they peel back those intellectual layers and filters. The pursuit of truth is the pursuit of God, which is the *tikun* for the sin of the first man and woman. Man added layers of reality to Creation, and history has been about the removal of those layers as much as possible.[5]

Simply, you need *Da'as* to recognize and connect to God. But not just any *Da'as*, but *this* kind:

> *If you want it as you do silver, and search after it like buried treasures, then you will understand fear of God—Da'as Elokim you will find.* (*Mishlei* 2:4)

There are two paths to *Da'as Elokim, Pardes* and *pain. Pardes* is the Torah route. The word means "orchard," but in this case it alludes to four levels of Torah

---

[5] See the Introduction.

learning, from the simplest to the sublime:

> There are four levels [of Torah learning], and their *roshei teivos*[6] spell *Pardes*. [The four levels are] *Pshat*, *Remez*, *Drush*, and *Sod*—Simple, Hint, Elucidation, and Secret. (*Sha'ar HaGilgulim*, Introduction 11)

All four levels can apply to any kind of Torah learning because just about every Torah concept has a simple meaning, a little more sophisticated level of meaning, a more *midrashic* type meaning, and *kabbalistic* understanding.

For example, most verses in the Torah can be understood simply as read.[7] *Rashi* and other commentators often add to that understanding by showing how words in the verse allude to deeper ideas. The *Midrash* provides a lot of the backstory to many verses while the *Gemora* elucidates verses for *halachic* purposes. It is the *Zohar* that reveals the *kabbalistic* inferences.

It is about getting to the *essence* of an idea because if it is a truth, then the essence will be a part of God, so-to-speak. God is a puzzle to mankind because He is so hidden, but every truth uncovered is another piece of the puzzle put into its place. The more pieces of the puzzle a

---

[6] Literally, *head letters*, that is, the first letter of each Hebrew word which is, *Peh, Raish, Samech,* and *Dalet*, which combined happened to spell *pardes*.

[7] See my book, *Kabbalah, Really?* for more details and examples of this.

person has, the more accurate their vision of God will be, as much as we are allowed to know it.

Not to worry. The vision of God we are allowed to perceive is so much more sophisticated than the average person can comprehend, at least at this stage of history. The most complicated secular knowledge only deals with the world in which they live, as vast as it may appear. The higher levels of knowledge of God go far beyond that.

That's why it is called *Da'as Elohim*. It is not only Godly knowledge, but knowledge *about* God. The spiritual world is to the light of God what the body is to the soul, a means of revelation. Therefore, the more you understand it, the more God becomes revealed to you.

Few people travel the *Pardes* route, or go far enough along its path. Each level of *Pardes* is rich with knowledge and clues to self-development that it is easy to get bogged down on one level or another. People spend entire lifetimes learning *Gemora* and its many commentaries and go no further, never entering into the essence of the ideas that they study day and night.

Knowledge on that level can change the way you act, but not necessarily who you are.[8] Learning new *halachah*

---

[8] The *Leshem* explains that this was also the difference between the first set of tablets, *Toras Atzilus*, and the second set, *Toras Beriyah*. It is impossible *not* to automatically become more spiritually refined when learning *Toras Atzilus (Sod)*, but a person has to work to change themself when learning only *Toras Beriyah*, as we see and experience everyday.

directs us how to *halachically* serve God, but only by looking at the heart of the *halachah*, which is what *Sod* does, will a person change on the inside as well. That is *true Da'as Elohim*.

But everyone needs *Da'as Elohim*, if only for the sake of *Tikun Olam*. When *Moshiach* comes, he will not only save the Jewish people, but those worthy from the nations of the world. For this reason, there is an alternative route, the path of pain and suffering.

Pain is humbling, and that is important. Humility is the key to *Da'as Elohim*, which is why Moshe *Rabbeinu* was not only a master of *Da'as Elohim*, but he was also the humblest person on the face of the earth.[9] Each made the other possible.

Because humility is not about thinking little of yourself. It is about being so objective in life that only the things that matter most to God matter most to you. As much as each of us matter to God, and we do, still, He has even more important things on His mind and agenda. If we're on His page, then egotism is just a big distraction and huge waste of energy.

If *Pardes* goes through a person as much as a person goes through *Pardes*, then this should be the automatic net result. If neither occurs, then pain should accomplish through the suffering of the body what *Pardes* is meant to accomplish through the mind.

---

[9] *Bamidbar* 12:3.

It is rare that a successful and confident person will also truly be humble. Possible, but rare.[10] This is why the *Gemora* says that Torah is more likely to come from the mouths of the poor,[11] if only because of their innate humility and limited amount of material distraction. It also says that secrets of life come as a gift to those who fear God, presumably for the same reason.[12]

Every pain is humbling because it makes a person confront their limitations. But it takes the right amount of pain for the right amount of time to make a person accept that, as clever and capable as they are, they are subservient to a higher power.

If they're smart, the suffering person will realize from the beginning that the higher power is God Himself, and immediately begin to change their life accordingly. They'll figure out early that God has many ways to execute His will, especially through the actions of people, and they won't be fooled by the power His "messengers" seem to assume to have. They'll see God as the true origin of their pain.

If they're not so smart, they may have to learn the truth in stages. After all, the purpose of life is to use our free will to choose good over evil, and it isn't much of a free will choice if we are compelled to choose the right way by

---

[10] Rebi Yehudah *HaNasi* (*Kesuvos* 104a) and Rebi Elazar *ben* Charsum (*Yoma* 35b) were a couple of exceptions.
[11] *Nedarim* 81a.
[12] *Niddah* 20b.

what we are going through.

Unless, of course, like Pharaoh back in Moshe's time, the person holds out on the truth as long as their ego will let them. If they're going to abuse their privilege of free will, then eventually they will lose their privilege of free will, and the pain will break them. The *hester panim*, the *histalkus* of Divine light will become very intense, like during the Holocaust.

But even the Holocaust led to something positive. People have argued about whether or not officially getting back the land of Israel in 1948 was part of the final redemption or not, but it is hard to argue that it wasn't a great thing for the Jewish people. It is also hard to argue (though some try to) that it would have happened when it did had not the Holocaust first occurred.

Why? Because every *histalkus* does not only leave behind something important necessary for the next stage of Creation. *Histalkus* is also another name for the most important part of rectifying Creation of which we are supposed to be a main part. It is called *Aliyas M"N,* and it will take a separate chapter to explain it.

four

Everyday people go about their lives oblivious to their digestive system. If they don't feel hungry or have an upset stomach, they ignore the very internal system that is in a large part responsible for keeping them alive 24/7. Out of sight, out of mind.

Smart people don't wait for problems to begin to be reminded of the need to maintain health. They use preventative medicine to learn in advance about how they need to live to keep living for as long as they can. They don't take their body's system for granted so they can use it to their best advantage.

The same thing is true about life. The average person gets up each day to perform certain activities they believe they need to do to make it to the next day, and the day after that, etc. They don't even necessarily know why, but that is what they have learned to do growing up in the world they live in.

They only start to ask questions when things do not go as hoped. They only question the system if they find cracks in its logic. They may feel powerless to change very much, but at least they have become aware of the need for change, and the courage to wonder what life is *really* about…on a deeper level.

It's like drinking water. Everyone knows it's important to drink water, but finding out why makes it easier to re-member to drink it each day, and more of it. For some, drinking a specific amount of water each day is even like taking a daily indispensable lifesaving medication. All of a sudden, something that is easily overlooked is no longer taken for granted.

Holy sparks are like that. In Hebrew, they are called *nitzotzei kedushah*, and not only do they keep us alive, but we build our portion in the World to Come with them. Isn't that enough reason to know what they are and what we're supposed to do with them?

They have a very long history, longer than our own. *Nitzotzei kedushah* originated before Creation, the result of a Divinely-orchestrated cataclysmic event (*Sheviras HaKeilim*) that laid the foundation for the world we know and inhabit.[1] They are, basically, individual sparks of God's

---

[1] See my book, *Highest Knowledge Ever* for a more detailed explana-tion.

infinite light (a miracle of life) with which God created the world and maintains it.

Nothing yet has indicated the challenge of life or the opportunity of man. For that we need to introduce another concept known from *Kabbalah* as the *Klipos,* the basis of evil in the world. They spiritually desensitize a person so that their *yetzer hara* can have a stronger influence over their actions and cause them to sin.

The *Klipos* can work through people or situations by preying on a person's spiritual vulnerabilities. A person who does not know about the *Klipos* and certainly one who does not take their *yetzer hara* seriously has lost the fight before it even began. As the *Ramchal* warned, if a person does not feel constantly at spiritual war with the *yetzer hara/Klipos,* then they have already lost the battle.

But what does this have to do with holy sparks? This:

When holiness (i.e., holy sparks) which is life, enters their domain (the *Klipos)*, they are nourished from it. They feed off [the holiness] because it is impossible for a holy soul to be cut off from its Holy Source… He (God) sends light, causing a flow of [spiritual] nourishment to those souls within the *Klipos,* and it is from this light that the *Klipos* also feed. (*Sha'ar HaGilgulim*, Introduction 15)

We need to eat to survive, and the *Klipos* need to eat to survive. We consume food to access the life-sustaining holiness of holy sparks inside it, and the *Klipos* cause people to sin in order to access the life-sustaining holiness within the souls among them. But *we* consume sparks so that we can live and do good and eventually destroy the *Klipos*. *They* consume them so that they can live and do evil, and eventually destroy good.

Hence the war. It's what results when two sides want the same thing and sharing is not in the cards. The terrifying thing, as the *Ramchal* points out, is how the good side knows little of the war while the *Klipos* live to fight it. While the average person casually learns Torah and performs *mitzvos* because that is their obligation and what they are used to doing, the *Klipos* work with abandon to get people to sin and steal their holiness.

Hence all the moral corruption in the world.

Hence all the wars throughout history.

Because it is not only an issue of an ongoing spiritual war with serious physical ramifications. It is primarily about *Tikun Olam*—World Rectification. This means all the *nitzotzei kedushah* out of the *Klipos*, the complete end of all evil,[2] and the completion of all of this by a certain date in history.[3] And nothing makes a battle more intense than a time limit on fighting it.

It's all about *aliyas M"N*, which stands for two Aramaic words, *Mein Nukvin*. They translate as "female waters,"

---

[2] *Sha'ar HaGilgulim*, Introduction 20.
[3] *Sanhedrin* 97a, 98a, and many other sources.

but they refer to the *nitzotzei kedushah* which we are expected to elevate to their spiritual source above. We do that best by learning Torah and performing *mitzvos*.

It's like gasoline in a car. An idle car burns no fuel. But if you drive it, the engine combusts the fuel, uses the energy, and then returns it to the universe in a different form. The more intense (faster) the drive, the faster the fuel is used up and returned to the universe.

Similarly, it takes fuel to act, and the more intensely you act, the faster you will burn that fuel and require more. It may seem like food is the source of that energy, but in truth it is the sparks within the food that give us what we need to live and accomplish. The more we live and accomplish, the more sparks we will need.

Live, *how*? Accomplish, *what*?

Even the secular world uses terms like "living dead." It acknowledges that physical life alone is not enough, and even becomes meaningless when the *quality of life* is very low. This is why many people over the ages have resorted to voluntarily ending their lives when they believed that physical life alone was not sufficient reason to continue living.

This of course has sparked many life-and-death debates about what constitutes true *quality of life*. But those debates end at the door of the *Shulchan Aruch*, which explicitly explains when it is permissible according to God to pull the plug on *physical* life. As to quality of life, the *Gemora* declares that "evil people, even while alive are considered dead…and righteous people, even after they have died are considered alive."[4]

The truth is, the *Gemora* is just echoing what the Torah long ago taught in no uncertain terms:

This day, I call upon the Heaven and the Earth as witnesses [that I have warned] you: I have set before you life and death, the blessing and the curse. Choose life, so that you and your offspring will live… (Devarim 30:19)

From the Torah it is clear that death here is not *physical* death, but *spiritual* death. And it is clear from what comes before this verse and after it that spiritual death means a Torah-less life. The Torah is saying, "Don't just choose to *physically* live. Choose to *spiritually* live as well, and really be alive."

Live…*a Torah life.*

Accomplish…*spiritual greatness.*

This means that a person can use up more sparks and better rectify Creation by a single spiritual act with *mesiras Nefesh*—self-sacrifice, than someone who runs for hours with everything they have. The runner will have physically sweat a lot more, but the *mitzvah* doer will have spiritually sweat a lot more, and that matters more in God's world.

---

[4] *Brochos* 18a.

Therefore, if enough people did enough *mitzvos* with enough *mesiras Nefesh* as per the Design schedule for creation and redemption, we would peacefully and joyously phase into the Messianic Era. The *Gemora* calls this approach *Achishenah*—Hastened,[5] because we would quickly strip the *Klipos* of all *nitzotzim* and cause their destruction earlier than later.

The problem arises when it does not happen this way, when *histalkus* and *aliyas M"N* is not only the result of Torah and *mitzvos*. What happens when the deadline for a redemption approaches and too many sparks remain in the *Klipos,* and not enough effort is being made to get them out on time?

This:

At that time [after the destruction of the Second Temple], sin increased and strengthened the *Klipos.* Man's actions lost the power to separate sparks from the kings;[6] they could no longer elevate *Mein Nukvin* (sparks)…Not only this, but even the *Mein Nukvin* from *Imma Ila'a*[7] returned and descended because

---

[5] *Sanhedrin* 98a.

[6] That is, from the combination of good and evil that resulted from the destruction of the pre-Creation *sefiros* whose names are taken from the kings of Edom mentioned at the end of *Parashas Vayishlach.*

[7] The level of *Binah* in the *sefiros,* which is a much higher source of sparks.

of the sins of the generation into the depths of the *Klipos,* combining with them like in the beginning.[8] This is the *sod* of [the verse], *"your mother was sent away for your sins."*[9] Consequently, the world was going to be destroyed, and it became necessary for them (the Ten Martyrs) to be killed *Al Kiddush Hashem.*[10] As a result, their souls were able to elevate *M"N* like in the beginning… (*Sha'ar Ma'amrei Rashb"i, Pekuday,* p. 167)

The point is, for the sake of the perfection of Creation and fulfillment of God's purpose in making it, sparks are going to be elevated no matter *what,* either *because* of us, or *through* us. We're going to elevate our quota of sparks either the *Pardes* route—*because of us*—or the *suffering* route—*through us*, and we, with our power of free will, get to decide which one.

It certainly seems like a no-brainer, or would if life

---

[8] Not only did we not elevate the sparks still waiting to be rectified, but we even reversed some of the earlier rectification by causing sparks from *Binah* to return to the *Klipos*, greatly strengthening the hand of evil.

[9] *Yeshayahu* 50:1. That is, the *nitzotzim* of *Imma* (mother) fell down into the *Klipos*.

[10] Sanctifying God's Name. The more a person suffers and nevertheless holds on to their faith in God, the greater a testimony it is to His existence. This is the most powerful way to elevate sparks, and it becomes necessary when we do not elevate them sufficiently sanctifying His Name through Torah and *mitzvos*.

were more straightforward. But when has life ever really been straightforward, starting with the first mistake man ever made when he ate the forbidden fruit of the *Aitz HaDa'as Tov v'Ra?* The warning was as straightforward as it gets—eat and you die—and yet Adam and Chava ate anyhow.

And they ate despite advance warning that they would:

> This is what the verse says in *Tehillim* 66:5: *"Go and see the deeds of God, awesome in His pretext— allilah—toward mankind."* Rebi Yehoshua *ben* Korchah said: "Even the awesome things You bring upon us You bring through pretext." Come and see how when The Holy One, Blessed is He, created the world He made the Angel of Death on the first day...[Yet] Adam wasn't created until the sixth [day], and was blamed for bringing death to the world as a pretext, as it says, *"On the day that you eat of it you shall certainly die"* (*Bereishis* 2:17). This is similar to someone who wants to divorce his wife and went home with a *get*.[11] He came home with the *get* in hand but wanted a pretext to give it to her. He told her, "Mix my cup so I can drink."[12] She made his drink and as

---

[11] A divorce document.

[12] They used to drink strong wine that required water to be added before drinking.

he took it from her he said, "Here is your *get*."

She asked him, "What did I do wrong?"

He told her, "Leave my house because you made me a lukewarm drink."

So she said to him, "You already knew that I would make you a lukewarm drink that you wrote a *get* and came with it in hand?"

Likewise, Adam said before The Holy One, Blessed is He, "For two thousand years before You created Your world the Torah was a nursling with You, as it says, *'I was a nursling beside Him, and I was [His] delight every day'* (*Mishlei* 30:8). And yet it says, *'This is the law of a person when he dies in a tent'* (*Bamidbar* 19:14). If you had not arranged for people to die, would You have written this? Rather, You want to blame it on me as a pretext." (*Tanchuma, Vayaishev* 4)

So much for free will and the ability to choose the non-painful path to rectification! It just seems sometimes as if God insists upon *aliyas M"N* happening *through us* instead of *because of us*, even manipulating history to make it so. If the first man, who didn't even have a *yetzer hara* yet, could not outsmart history, how can we be expected to *with* a *yetzer hara*?

Maybe we're not. Maybe we haven't yet gone deep enough into the mechanics of history to see an even bigger picture than the one we have seen so far. It doesn't mean

that we're wrong, just not fully there, or at least as fully
there as we are allowed to be. After all, we *are* talking
about God, *infinite* God, whose idea of good goes far beyond any level of good we so far comprehend.

Nevertheless, there may be room to go a little further,
a little higher.

five

oshe *Rabbeinu* first learned about the bigger big picture during his first forty days on *Har Sinai.* The *Gemora* fills us in on what happened:

When Moshe ascended to the Heaven he found The Holy One, Blessed is He, sitting and tying crowns on to letters. He said to Him, "Master of the World! Why are You doing this?"

God answered him, "There will be a man in the future after many generations and Akiva *ben* Yosef will be his name. He will elucidate every point and mound of law."

"Master of the Universe, show him to me."

"Turn around," God told him.

He turned around and [entered the future.] He sat at the back of eight rows [of a class Rebi Akiva was teaching]. When Moshe did not recognize what they were discussing he became distressed until a student asked, "Rebi, where did you learn that?"

Rebi Akiva answered them, "It is a *halachah* from Moshe from Mt. Sinai."

His (Moshe's) mind became settled and he returned to The Holy One, Blessed is He. He said to Him, "Master of the Universe! You have someone like that and You want to give the Torah through me?!"

God answered him, "Quiet! *Alah b'machshavah lefanai*—It went up in My mind before Me!"

So he said to Him, "Master of the Universe, you showed me his Torah, now show me his reward!"

He told him [again], "Turn around."

He turned around and saw them weighing his flesh in the market place and [horrified] he exclaimed, "Master of the Universe! This is Torah and this is its reward?!"

He answered [again], "Quiet! *Alah b'machshavah lefanai!*" (*Menachos* 29b)

It's a troubling *Gemora* on the level of *Pshat, Remez,* and *Drush*, each of which deal with the story as is. It is only on the level of *Sod* that a door is opened somewhat to an incredible world of understanding of everything, the *bigger* big picture.

Let's cut to the chase (because the full story takes years and volumes to properly tell). *Machshavah* is the *Moach Stima'a* of *Adam Kadmon* where *birrur*—separation—occurred between the holy and less holy lights to make Creation and the *Klipos*. *Alah* is what the lights did to ascend to the *Moach Stima'a* for *birrur* after *Sheviras HaKeilim* for *birrur*.

That's why God told Moshe, "Quiet!" He wasn't telling him to stop talking. He was answering his question about Rebi Akiva. God was explaining to Moshe that the answer he needed was too sublime to be expressed in words, something to do with the primordial ascension and separation of sparks, so he'd have to wait until he got to a point where he could learn it without the need for words.

History is like a tree. Just like you can only see the part of the tree that is above ground, similarly we can only see history since Creation. But just as the most crucial answers about the tree's life are hidden below ground, likewise are the most crucial answers about history before Creation.

However, unlike with respect to a tree, whose roots can be dug up and examined, pre-Creation is completely inaccessible to man unless God tells us about it, which he did. Moshe *Rabbeinu* may not yet have known it at the *beginning* of the forty years, which is when the incident above occurred. But he certainly knew all about it by the time he left Har Sinai two years later, and certainly when he died on *Har Nevo*.[1] It's what Rebi Shimon *bar* Yochai later revealed as part of the *Zohar*.

But what the *Rashb"i* really did was detail what the prophets Yeshayahu and Yechezkel long before him had already alluded to, *Ma'aseh Merkavah*—the Work of the Chariot. As the Jewish people entered exile for the first time in history since moving into *Eretz Yisroel,* and after witnessing what they had thought was the impossible destruction of the First Temple, they were reassured with new knowledge of a *bigger* big picture.

Thanks to the *Rashb"i* and later day *kabbalists* like Rabbi Moshe Cordovero and especially the *Arizal*, we have a lot of those details. Not most of them, since most of that knowledge still remains far beyond human grasp and words, but enough of them to get a *better* picture of the *bigger* picture.

Now, the thing about free will is that you don't have to actually accomplish what you plan to be acknowledged for it. If you run to help someone who insists they don't need your help, you are rewarded for having helped them anyhow even if you can't.[2] What a person wills given what life throws at them is in their control. What that will ends up doing is not.

---

[1] *Nevo* is spelled *Nun-Bais-Vav*, which is *Nun,* as in the *Nun Sha'arei Binah*—Fifty Gates of Understanding—in it. He had been born with the forty-nine of the fifty gates (*Nedarim* 21b), and was given the fiftieth at death on the mountain.

[2] *Brochos* 6a.

The rabbis phrased it like this:

All is in the hands of Heaven except the fear of Heaven. (*Brochos* 34b)

On a simple level this means that Heaven controls everything except our fear of Heaven, which most people understand to mean our *fear of punishment*. A person can choose to see that Heaven takes note of everything we do, evaluates our actions, rewards us for the good and punishes us for the bad…even if we can't see how or when.

But they didn't say fear of consequence for a reason. Maybe they were hinting that we can choose to understand why everything is in the hands of Heaven by increasing our awareness of what Heaven is and how it works. Fear in this sense being more a sense of awe, what everyone gets when they take the time to learn, understand, and appreciate *Ma'aseh Merkavah*.

Maybe this was the deeper message to Chizkiah *HaMelech* who tried to second guess God. The righteous king had a prophecy that he would father an evil son, so he avoided marriage altogether, not an easy thing to personally do especially as king.

Heaven's response to his seemingly noble act:

What did The Holy One, Blessed is He, do? He brought suffering to Chizkiah and told Yeshayahu, *"Go and visit the sick"*…

"Why do I deserve such a severe punishment?" Chizkiah asked.

"Because," answered Yeshayahu, "you did not have children."

"But I saw through prophecy that I would have an evil child!"

"What business do you have with *kavshei Rachmana*—the mysteries of God?" (*Brochos* 10a)

The *Gemora* goes on to say that Chizkiah not only almost died fifteen years early, but he almost lost his portion in the World to Come as well. But as Chizkiah pointed out, his was an unusually severe punishment for the sin committed, especially given his intention.

So Yeshayahu explained that it wasn't just his ignoring of such a fundamental *mitzvah* as procreation, but it also had to do with his playing God. Because that is what a person does when they second guess God, because they act as if they know better than God does, and that is an aspect of idol worship.

But again, perhaps there is a deeper point here. Maybe what Yeshayahu was really telling Chizkiah is:

If you leave the ways of God a mystery, then you have no business questioning them. But if you take the time to understand the *bigger* big picture, then you will find that there really is no need to second guess God. It will be a lot easier to stay with the program even when the results are the *opposite* of what you intended.

In other words, there is Divine method to the Divine madness, which is really only madness to us, which is not saying a whole lot. God is infinitely wise, and we are but teensy finite beings by comparison. Somehow at some point mankind made the audacious, and really quite ridiculous assumption that *His* wisdom should be subject to ours. Are people ever in for a shock.

The question is not, why doesn't more of God's plan make sense to us? The question is, how do we even understand anything about it? Like we say in *Shemonah Esrai*, human understanding is a great gift, and the thing about a gift is that you only get as much of it as the giver decides to give.

But that's okay. We don't need to understand every last detail of God's plan for Creation, or even just most of them. We just need to know enough of them to be able to see that He is in control, everything is for our good, and we really have no reason *not* to trust Him for the process. If we don't, that's on us because it means that we haven't done our homework sufficiently, or worked hard enough to keep our egos at bay.

So what *is* the bigger picture?

It's actually detailed in the *Zohar*, specifically in *Idra Rabba, Idra Zuta*, and *Sifri D'Tzniusa*. But unless you are already a certified *kabbalist*, you won't understand a word.

Oh, and you need to be fluent in Aramaic as well, and specifically the Aramaic used by the *Zohar*, which is a little different than the one used by the *Gemora*.

Fortunately, there have been some *kabbalists* along the way who have understood the *Zohar* enough to explain it in more graspable terms. Books have been written, *drushim* have been given, and teachers have been teaching. But still, unless a person makes the effort and takes the time to learn them well, their explanations will also remain beyond comprehension.

And there is this as well. Dovid *HaMelech* told us that *"the secrets of God go to those who fear Him."*[3] God may not be particular about who learns math or algebra, but He is about who gets to see His secrets of Creation. It's one thing to read the words and comprehend their meaning, but it something very different to *feel* their reality to the point of being impacted by them.

How do you know if you are? Because those secrets were shared for only one purpose. In fact, the entire Torah was given to us for that same purpose. And the truth be known, everything was created just for this purpose, and if a person sees any of it and does not feel compelled to contribute to the fulfillment of that purpose, then they know that God has kept them on the outside.

Because as smart as we are, and people can be *really* smart, we still need *siyata D'Shemaya*—Heavenly help—

---

3 *Tehillim* 25:14.

when it comes to connecting to truth, which is really connecting to God. All relationships are two-way, and if a person is not prepared to share themself with God, then why should God share Himself with them? *Chitzonius*[4] is available to everyone, but *Penimius*[5] is only for those who are part of God's inside circle.

It makes sense. The bigger big picture explains that everything God has ever done and will ever do as far as man is concerned has been for the sake of revelation. The entire system, phenomenally intricate and complicated, was built and is maintained to make possible God's revelation to something else. If a person tries to help with this then they are in synch with God. If not, then they are missing the entire point of existence.

The revelation of God is not a side point. It is the *only* point. It may not happen immediately, but it will happen eventually, God will see to it. We may not be able to see now how what is happening will lead to it, but we will at some time in the future. That's when we will be able to have God show us how what we perceived as Divine madness had been in fact the most logical path, given its final destination.

But why wait? Why not sneak a peek now while it still

---

[4] External knowledge that deals with the physical world, like secular studies.

[5] Internal knowledge, which is knowledge that speaks from the soul to the soul.

bothers us to see so much injustice and falsehood in the world, all on God's watch? If God is willing to de-mystify Himself somewhat, who are we to say no, at least if we're going to complain about negative outcomes and second guess His judgments?

It's decision time. If you now feel that you know enough to do neither, but to instead just trust God no matter what makes sense, then you can skip the next chapter. You probably won't skip it anyhow, but that's a good thing because it will help you realize that you didn't really understand as much as you thought you had, or needed to.

six

It is not unusual for people traveling short distances to not notice or care about one another. More than likely if you got on a city bus and, sitting down next to a complete stranger, you asked them their name, they would probably think you were creepy.

On the other hand, it is hard *not* to get to know a person you are traveling with for a much longer period of time, like on an overseas flight for example, at least someone in your row. Then it seems stranger if you insist on remaining strangers.

Yet, how many people truly know *themselves*, their travel partner for life? They just assume they do. This is why most people go through life never really understanding who they are. This is why most people go through life never really understanding what they need or could accomplish in life.

No wonder the depression rate is so high. One would think that, statistically, the rate should be higher among people lacking the financial means to live a decent life. Even though people like to say that money can't buy happiness, they pursue it and live as if it can.

The cold, hard truth is that very often people with less materialism in life are happier than people with more. This is because happiness is not something you can fake to yourself, and though we were made to love the material world, we were also built to only have happiness from being who we truly are in essence.

That was simple long before we started paying attention to the rest of the world. Before then, we just *were*. We hadn't yet become familiar with societal norms because we hadn't yet become familiar with society. Life was pretty automated at that point.

The first thing to steal our show was the *yetzer hara*. The *yetzer hara* is survival instinct on steroids. All of a sudden and from an early age, everything that catches our attention is something we need and want and, apparently, already belongs to us even if it doesn't. If we don't get it, the world will know about it in no uncertain terms.

A little older and a little smarter, we learn by necessity to replace some of our brawn with brains. Seeing how crowded the world is, how many people want the same things that we do, and how much more powerful some people are, we realize that cleverness, and even deceit to some degree, can serve us better in the long run.

But it seems as if the more we let society into our lives, the more we leave ourselves out. The thing we need most in life to feel happy, and that requires self-validation. But too often, in order to survive, people hand the power of self-validation to others. This forces them to live up to the standards of others and become sad when they don't…even though they really are quite good.

Some sense this and go soul-searching. The only question is if they have the right guide and look in the correct place because there are plenty of wrong directions to go. Sometimes good only looks good compared to bad. But next to great, good may look a lot less good and end up being a big waste of life.

Pain helps with that, a lot. If we only knew how many happy people are that way because they found themselves through suffering. Religion like anything else can be an opium if approached only as a painkiller. But God is the essential truth a person comes to once they come to their essential self, and pain can certainly help that process.

It really does not require too much explanation why, but here is some nonetheless.

To begin with, pain is an attention grabber. It's like someone snapping their fingers in front of our faces while we are in a trance. Whatever was fighting for our attention before, whatever we focused on prior to the pain, all of it gets pushed to the back burner while we give our undivided attention to our pain.

We don't want to, but we have to. Our bodies demand it. Our brains command it. Even if we already know that the pain poses no immediate threat, still pain goes after us as if there is. It takes time before a person can will their attention away from their pain, and some never can because some pains just can't be vetoed.

There is a true story of a woman who was diagnosed with and was dying from brain cancer. On a visit from the shul rabbi, she told him that she was grateful to God for her cancer because, she told the *Rav*, "Before I had it I didn't know what life was about. Now I do."

The *rav* assumed that she didn't really mean what she said, but was just making peace with her critical situation. But against his better judgment, he asked her, "If you had the chance to do it all again, would you?" probably regretting every word once they came out of his mouth.

To his surprise and awe, the woman didn't even have to think about it. She answered without thinking twice, *"Yes, because now I know what life is about."* Apparently she had decided already that a short, even painful life full of meaning is better than a longer one that lacks it.

But what did she really learn that she did not know before? Ironically, it's what we go in search of every *Yom Kippur* if you know what you're looking for.

After all, what are we trying to prove on *Yom Kippur* with all of our *inu'im*,[1] dovening the whole day with more

---

[1] Afflictions, the five pleasures we abstain from on *Yom Kippur*.

intention than we do the rest of the year, and to whom? God? Doesn't He already know our outcome on *Yom Kippur* before we even start the day? He's above time, remember?

We're there on *Yom Kippur*, in principle, to answer one question, and we're there to answer it specifically for ourselves. The question? *Who are we really*? Who are we in essence? What is the main thing we want in life, and *from* life? In other words, what is our *essential* will, something we tend to lose track of in life if a person ever knew it in the first place?

How can *Yom Kippur* help with that? It depends. If a person is basically satisfied with who they are when they go into *Yom Kippur* more than likely that is how they will come out of *Yom Kippur*. If they feel self-satisfied they will assume, and dangerously so, that God is also happy with them, especially if they fasted, came to *shul*, and did their time. They will not be any more in touch with themself than they were before.

But if a person goes into *Yom Kippur* to connect to God on the highest level possible, they will feel the distance between themself and God. As they try to pray with complete sincerity to connect to God, as if in a personal conversation with Him, they will feel how distant they are from that level of *dveikus*.[2]

If the person pushes further, they will confront what

---

[2] Clinging to God.

it is about them that blocks them from pursuing God, loving God, and trying to connect to Him regularly. When we search for our sincerity we come closer to who we are in essence. It is only called sincerity when what we say or do comes from our essential being, or essential *ratzon*—will, not from someone else we evolved into to satisfy the misguided demands of others.

Here's the problem. Once upon a time, while man was still free of an onboard *yetzer hara* there was no mistaking who was in charge and who was responsible for everything. With the birth of Kayin and Hevel, that changed. From that point onward, mankind had an internal *yetzer hara* that shares the same brain with the *yetzer tov*.

It makes life very confusing. How do you know who's talking? How do you know if a command comes from the *yetzer tov* or the *yetzer hara*? And what about the people who don't even know or believe they have a *yetzer hara*? What happens to them?

It's a problem. If a person does not believe they have a *yetzer hara* they will be corrupt. It's inevitable. There will be many times throughout their lives when they are going to want something illicit and find ways to get it. It's much harder to say no to ourselves than it is to say it to others, at least when a person lacks a conscience.

Such people will also deny themselves the opportunity to get to the core being. The layers added over the years will be considered part and parcel of who they are, and they have to learn to live with it. If you don't think something is broke, why would you even consider fixing it?

But if a person lives with the reality that they have a *yetzer hara*, and that they are not it, then they can achieve separation. They know who the enemy is and can develop a battle strategy to keep it at bay and, if they are really clever, harness its power for good.

At the very least, and it is not least at all, such a person has a chance to find themself in essence—*and be it*. There is no greater sense of completion in life, no greater sense of accomplishment, and certainly no greater joy than being exactly who we are in essence.

The following *middos* (traits) help a person to achieve separation from the *yetzer hara*, and to measure how close they are to being who they really are. Because, they are examples of who we *all* are in essence, and to the extent that they resonate on a scale between 1 (a little) and 10 (a lot) with you, that is the extent to which you are being you. This is how the soul thinks:

Want to Be Special

Special here means using your personal abilities to accomplish as much as you can, and not just accepting mediocrity.

Love God

We were created to love. It is the most natural thing to do, like loving parents. We are happiest when we feel love for God and, more importantly, His love back to us.

Love Torah & Understanding Truth

The greatest pleasure a soul has is being connected to truth, because a soul itself is all truth, and it is like going home. Most important of all is that the "seal of God" is truth, so truth itself connects a person to God.

Generous and Kind

The image of God in which we were made refers to our soul, and we best exhibit it through generosity and kindness to others. This is why God won't forgive a sin on *Yom Kippur* between two people unless the damaged person first forgives the damager. Our relations with others reveal our Godliness and ability to connect to God.

Disciplined

When the going gets tough, the tough get going. The question is, what does it mean to be tough in this sense? It means appreciating life and the opportunity to get important and meaningful things done in whatever time we may be blessed to have. No one is really lazy, just unfocused or unappreciative of the opportunity they have.

Love to Pray

This is not an easy one for many people, but it would be if they really believed they were talking *with* God, as opposed to only *to* Him. But what people who do enjoy praying have found out is that once you get into *tefillah*, you start to feel as if God is right there with you, because He is. It's an incredible feeling that makes prayer so entrancing.

Modest

One of the most accurate signs that society is headed by the *yetzer hara* is the lack of modesty. The Torah emphasizes modest behavior as a matter of self-dignity, to emphasize the preciousness and holiness of the soul inside the body. Just as we wrap valuable items in respectable packaging, we do the same for our souls and bodies, which can also become holy as a result

Despise Lewdness

The *Zohar* says that you can tell what a person is like by how they speak. How much more so is this true by the way a person carries themselves in public and by what entertains them. The body is not concerned about acting like an animal because it is not much different. But such behavior is not only beneath the soul, it disgusts it.

Not Materialistic

The general rule is, the less spiritual a person is, the more they tend to compensate with material pleasures. Everyone wants to feel real and alive, and we do that best when living like a soul, as Ya'akov *Avinu* did. A person out of touch with their spiritual side is forced to depend upon temporal physical pleasures to make them feel as if they exist, an Eisav-like approach to life.

Hate Evil

Evil takes many forms, but at its root it is the absence of Divine light in the world. To love God is to hate evil, and all that it causes, like injustice, etc.

Appreciative

The soul, unlike the body, has no sense of entitlement. It is completely selfless, so it tends to count its blessings and be grateful for them.

The list can go on and on, but the idea is, the more a person identifies with such positive traits, the greater the separation they can achieve from their *yetzer hara*. It won't happen immediately, or even easily, but even small steps in this direction are noticeable, encouraging, and very uplifting.

But you can expect a fight. The *yetzer hara* does not give in easily and will fight back. It can even take revenge, in a manner of speaking, counteracting your drive for spiritual growth with obstacles to it. That's its job, to create spiritual challenge so that you can use your God-given ability of free will to choose to be free of the *yetzer hara*.

As the *Gemora* says, the difference between a *tzaddik* and *rasha* (evil person) is not whether they fall or not. *Tzaddikim* fall too, and sometimes often. As Shlomo *HaMelech* wrote:

> *For there is no righteous man on earth who does good and does not sin.* (*Koheles* 7:20)

A *rasha* however only has to spiritually fall once and not get up, while a *tzaddik* keeps getting up no matter how many times they fall. They know that though all results in life are in the hands of Heaven, their fear of God is theirs to develop and maintain...until their dying day.

The most important part? Having made the separation between your essential self and your *yetzer hara*, you can be yourself, your true self. When the *yetzer hara* approaches you, you'll be able to recognize it as the *yetzer hara*, and exclude it from the decision making process.

There is no underestimating the importance of such an accomplishment in life, or of how that is the true definition of success in life. We're not here to become business people, musicians, educators, etc. Those are all just different means to one end: the essential *you*.

Sometimes we only find things in life by actually creating them. Sometimes they already exist, and we just have to reveal them. Your essential self falls into the second category, and that's good news. The difficult part is pulling back the layers to reveal it, and that will depend upon how tightly covered your essential self has become over the years.

It's like the difference between finding something under a stack of papers, or having to dig it out after a hurricane has passed through. If a person has grown up with an emphasis on self-honesty and appreciation of truth, finding their essential self may only be a matter of rearranging priorities.

But if a person has lived a life weak on moral principles and the idea that they need to be something they are not, or should never be, getting to the bottom of themself can be like pulling back the remains of a collapsed building to get to what is buried inside. No wonder some people never try and give up instead.

But as the *Gemora* says, "Someone who comes to purify themself, they help them."[3] This means that if a person takes a few steps in the right direction, God will take even bigger steps on their behalf. *Teshuvah* is a miracle, and is only possible with Heavenly help, which God is only too willing to give to the person who is willing to try.

---

[3] *Yoma* 38a.

seven

There is another side to the pain story. God never makes a person suffer for no good reason, but often times He accomplishes two purposes with one illness.

We already saw an example of this[1] regarding Chizkiah *HaMelech* and Yeshayahu *HaNavi*:

Rav Hamnuna said: What does the verse, *"Who is like the wise man, and who knows the interpretation—pesher—of the matter"* (*Koheles* 8:1) mean? It means, who is like The Holy One, Blessed be He, Who knows how to bring about a compromise—*peshara*—between two righteous individuals, Chizkiah and

---

[1] See Chapter 5.

Yeshayahu [who disagreed over which of them should go to the other]. Chizkiah said: "Let Yeshayahu come to me like Eliyahu who went to Achav"…Yeshayahu said: "Let Chizkiah come to me, like Yehoram *ben* Achav who went to Elisha." What did The Holy One, Blessed is He, do? He brought suffering to Chizkiah and told Yeshayahu, "Go and visit the sick"… (*Brochos* 10a)

As the *Gemora* explains, Chizkiah had his own reason to become deathly ill, but God also used it as an excuse to bring two stubborn people together. In the next story that is also true, someone else's suffering gave a young man an opportunity to perform a great *mitzvah*, and change his own life in the process:

A few years ago, there was a young man in New York who was an outstanding *talmid chacham*, someone who at a young age was already deciding *halachah*, leading others, and showing signs of inner greatness. At a certain point, this young *talmid chacham* was tested by Rav Yochanan Wosner *Shlit"a*, the *Sqverer Dayan* and world-renowned *posek*. The young man was beyond exceptional. Rav Wosner, who is a very perceptive person, felt that there was something special going on, and asked the young man. "Could I please meet with your father?"

A few days later, Rav Yochanan Wosner met this

young *posek*'s father. "Can I ask you a question?" asked Rav Wosner in the middle of the conversation. "Was your son always like this? Was he always a diligent *masmid*? Did he always have such a clear understanding of the *sugyos*?"

"It is so interesting you ask," the father responded. "The truth is that *no*, my son was not always so focused, and he didn't always understand everything so easily."

"So what happened? What made him suddenly take off?" the *Rav* asked.

"About seven years ago my son was still in *yeshiva*. A big *yeshiva*. He was a wonderful *talmid* but not so special in learning, definitely not in the top of the *shiur*. One Thursday morning he was called up for *hagbah*[2] after *Krias HaTorah*.[3] My son went up and did what is called a reverse-*hagbah*—the *hagbah* that we only do on *Simchas Torah*.[4] Everyone was

---

[2] The lifting of a *Sefer Torah* for all to see just before returning it to the Ark.

[3] Torah reading.

[4] On all other occasions, the person raising up the *Sefer Torah* for all to see picks it up with the writing facing him, and then turns around for all those to see it. On *Simchas Torah*, the person lifting the *Sefer Torah* takes the handles of the Torah in opposite hands so that when he lifts it and straightens out his hands, the writing in the Torah is facing the congregation, and the back of the *Sefer Torah is* facing him.

shocked at first, and then the smiles and snickering began. Very soon, the reverse-*hagbah* became the talk of the *yeshiva*. Hilarious. Another one of his antics. The *Rosh Yeshivah*, who was also present, asked one of his *gabbaim* to call my son after breakfast. My son went into the *Rosh Yeshiva*'s office, who then asked him, 'Why did you do it?' He was not angry. He was simply bewildered. My son looked down at his shoes. He didn't want to tell at first, but after a few moments, he looked up and simply said, 'Does the *Rosh Yeshivah* remember who was called up for *shlishi*?[5] It was Yankele, the boy with a terrible stutter. He took five minutes to read the *brochah* before *shlishi* and another five minutes for the *brochah* after *shlishi*. I could see so many *buchurim*[6] trying to hold back frustrations and smiles, and I knew I had to think quickly. I had to find something that would divert everyone's attention so that no one would remember Yankele's *shlishi* and would only remember me. So I did a reverse-*hagbah*, and it worked. No one remembers *shlishi* any longer!' The *rosh yeshiva* started to cry. My son had shown that he had the sensitivity to be someone who people needed. And from that day on all the wellsprings of wisdom

---

[5] The third of three people called up on a Monday, Thursday, or *Shabbos Mincha* Torah reading.
[6] Young *yeshivah* students.

opened up to him."

The father wasn't necessarily saying that his son's success in Torah was the direct result of his great sensitivity towards others, and his willingness to embarrass himself to save others from shame. How could he know for sure, even if he believed it with all his heart?

But if it wasn't, then what a coincidence, which we do not believe in. Even if a person has a difficult time accepting that years of success in Torah can be tied to a single event in one's youth, they should have an equally difficult time dismissing the possibility. The timing is too uncanny, especially since the young man had not shown signs of greatness prior to his act of *mesiras Nefesh*.

Pain doesn't just change the life of the one suffering it. It also changes the lives of the people suffering through them. Even the *Rosh Yeshivah* who had heard his *talmid* stutter through his *brochah* was not nearly as moved by what happened as he was once his other *talmid* explained his actions.

The *Rosh Yeshivah* and his *talmid* had been years apart in age and wisdom, but at that time the student had become the teacher. And not just of his *Rosh Yeshivah*, but of all of those who have since read his story and taken it to heart. And to think that all of that merit can be tied back to a boy who could not say his Torah blessings clearly, something most can and take for granted.

Again, the boy with the stutter has his own *cheshbon*

with God as to why he has to put up with such a debilitating problem. But it is clear from the story and so many
others like it that personal suffering is not as personal as it
seems. What we go through in life, happy or sad, impacts
the lives of others around us, whether we know it or not.

There is another example of this idea in the Torah
itself here:

> *When you come to the land of Canaan which I am
> giving you as a possession, and I place a lesion of
> tzara'as in a house in the land of your possession...*
> (*Vayikra* 14:34)

It was [good] news that lesions of *tzara'as* will come
to them because the Amorites had hidden away treasures of gold inside the walls of their houses during
the entire forty years that the Jewish people were in
the desert. As a result of the lesion, the person will
have to demolish the house and find them. (*Rashi*)

There is nothing pleasant about *tzara'as*. It was like a
form of leprosy when on a person except that it came for
spiritual reasons, like speaking *loshon hara* for example.
First it appeared on the walls of the sinner's home, and if
they did not heed the Divine warning it appeared on their
clothing. If they persisted with the sin then it eventually
appeared on the person's skin.

The *halachos* of *tzara'as* and the *metzora* are many

and complicated. There might be limited physical pain, but the spiritual and emotional pain can be a lot. One thing is for certain: no one gets *tzara'as* without Divine reason, whether on their body, their clothing, or the walls of their house.

After all, if house *tzara'as* was only meant as a means to discover hidden treasures, God could have found a less disruptive way to reveal it. Finding the treasure did not mean the homeowner was free of all the *halachic* realities of *tzara'as* in a house. The good news *and* the bad news were both valid and real.

Like the New Yorker who tried to build a *succah* on his high rise balcony and was court-ordered to take it down. So he spoke to a gentile who owned the roof apartment in his building and made an actual contractual deal (the gentile insisted on it) to pay an exorbitant amount of money (and he insisted on this too) to build his *succah* on the roof for eight days.

But when he got there, he was quite dismayed to find that the roof was more like a garbage dump than a place to fulfill the *mitzvah* of *succah*. He had clearly been taken advantage of but at that point there was nothing to do but clean the place up and build his *succah*, which he did.

However, in the process of cleaning up he discovered a hidden stash of jewelry worth a king's ransom. After some investigation, it was found out that the jewels had belonged to an elderly man who had passed away years ago without leaving the jewelry to anyone. According to New

York, the jewels belonged to the one who found them.

The gentile on whose roof the jewels had been found of course contested the ruling. But it turned out that the contract that *he* had insisted writing, and by a top-dollar lawyer at the Jew's expense, actually gave the claim to the riches to the Jew. Nothing erases the bitter memory of suffering faster than a sweet ending to all of it.

It's ironic that such a story should be about a *succah*, given this one in the *Gemora*:

> [In the future, the gentiles will] say before Him: "Master of the Universe, give us [the Torah] and we will perform it."
>
> The Holy One, Blessed is He, [will] answer them: "Fools of the world! One who prepares on *Erev Shabbos* will eat on *Shabbos*, but one who did not prepare on *Erev Shabbos*, from what will he eat on *Shabbos*? [The opportunity for performing *mitzvos* has already passed, and it is now too late to ask to perform them.] Even so, I have an easy *mitzvah* [for you to fulfill], and it is called *succah*. Go and perform it."
>
> …And why [does God] call [*succah*] easy to fulfill? Because it involves no monetary loss. (*Avodah Zarah* 3a)

Perhaps once-upon-a-time and a very long time ago *Succos* was an inexpensive holiday. But in recent years *Suc-*

cos has become one of the more *expensive* holidays. It certainly cost the Jew in the story an arm-and-a-leg to build his *succah*, and would have had he not been blessed with amazing *Hashgochah Pratis* to find the jewels and have the contract imposed upon by the gentile businessman.

But maybe this was not a random act but the message of *succah* embodied in reality. A *succah* represents many things, but above all, it is a reminder of Who watches over the Jewish people and takes care of all our needs. And as *Chazal* teach, we specifically go into our *succos* during the cooler and rainier season of Fall, when most others leave their summer dwellings behind to emphasize this idea.

But as the *Gemora* says, Heaven does not help someone unless they take the first steps on their own.[7] They do not sanctify them a lot unless they first sanctify themself a little. Yes, we may have to pay some good money to build a good *succah*. But having done that God then finds ways to not only pay us back for our outlay, but even to give us more beyond it.

Perhaps that is why God will give the gentiles who ask for Torah in the future time the *mitzvah* of *succah*. It was really His answer to them:

You can't have Torah now, because Torah was about more than learning it and performing its *mitzvos*. It

---

[7] *Yoma* 38a.

was about doing all of that during a time in history when it did not always make sense to do so, and could even be painful to fulfill *mitzvos*. It is about developing and having *emunah*, faith in God and His process when it was possible and necessary to have it. It was about asking for Torah *before* you knew the reward for living by it, not *after* as you do now.

Ultimately, that is the difference between those who live by Torah and those who don't. The ones who keep the faith believe in that other side of the story of pain, even if they can't even see a hint to it. Believers know that our current lives are not the end of any story, just a specific part of it. They understand that Divine justice goes far beyond human experience, but that good *always* triumphs in the end.

In fact, we can even go further. If the *Zohar's* fascinating revelation of *gilgulim* (reincarnations) teaches us anything, it is that what happens to us in any given lifetime is influenced by what we have done throughout *all* of our lifetimes. The *Arizal's* amazing detailing of the information of the *Zohar* in his work *Sha'ar HaGilgulim* shows us somewhat how much this is true, and why.

The long and short of it is that we're here for only one reason, *tikun*. Though we have mentioned this in earlier chapters, we did not discuss it on this level. Until this point *tikun* has meant rectifying the mistakes of previous generations. Bringing the idea of *gilgulim* into the discussion means previous *generations* also means previous *lifetimes*.

It's a long and *kabbalistic* story, but the basic idea is like this. Even though it is possible to have up until four different souls in one body, everybody only has one essential soul that is uniquely theirs. It is the only one that they need to rectify by the time history and the chance to reincarnate comes to a close.

One soul, but *five* parts. And the five parts have five parts, as do those five parts, etc. We have all five parts from birth because they connect us to God and act as our personal conduit to life-sustaining Divine light. But gaining access to the levels above the one on which we are born, which means being able to use their level of light at will, depends upon having rectified the levels below it.

According to the *Zohar*, a person should rectify the entire lowest level of soul—*Nefesh*—by age fourteen. If they remain on spiritual track they can, potentially, rectify the entire next level—*Ruach*—by age twenty. If they succeed, then they will be able to work on their third level, *Neshamah*. If they succeed before leaving this world, they will not have to return anymore for their own rectification.[8] They're done.

But should they die having left levels of soul unrectified, then they will have to reincarnate to pick up where

---

[8] They can return to help others with their rectification process, and gain extra reward for doing so (*Sha'ar HaGilgulim*, Introduction 5).

they left off in a previous lifetime. Whatever they did rectify by death becomes off-limits, meaning that a future life cannot undo previous success. And once that happens, then they can no longer finish off the rest of their unrectified levels in the same lifetime, but lifetime by lifetime.

Needless to say, *gilgulim* make life a lot more interesting and complicated. Herod blinded Babba *ben* Buta,[9] so Rav Sheishes, his reincarnation, was born blind.[10] Eliyahu HaNavi wasn't born, but evolved from Pinchas.[11] Aharon reincarnated from Haran and had a chance to rectify his mistake by dying to stop the golden calf rather than pretending to go along with it.[12]

Among the many things this teaches us, one of them is that the answers to current troubles might not be in current lifetimes, but in previous ones. This may not be something that can be confirmed in any absolute way, but it is also something not to be dismissed out of hand.

On one hand, learning about something as *kabbalistic* as *gilgulim* seems like a luxury since there are so many other practical areas of Torah study to become immersed in. But on the other hand, it seems that such information is indispensable for getting through life's challenges and figuring out personal *tikun*.

---

9 *Bava Basra* 4b.
10 *Sha'ar HaGilgulim*, Introduction 4.
11 *Sha'ar HaGilgulim*, Introduction 32.
12 *Sha'ar HaGilgulim*, Introduction 33.

And just because a person is not currently suffering doesn't mean that they don't need such information and insights. On the contrary, they may need it even more! After thousands of years and hundreds of generations, it is clear how easy it is to think you're walking the right path in life and miss it altogether. People only *think* they know who they are, but how many truly know themselves to their core?

Find and walk the correct path, and the pot of gold you'll find at the end of the journey is you, the *essential* you.

eight

ind over matter: if you don't *mind*, it doesn't *matter*. It has been said that God made sports to stop the pogroms. If they weren't busy killing each other or paying to watch it, they'd be killing Jews instead.

It might have been said tongue-in-check, but there is truth to it. The beatings that people are prepared to take and the aggression that they put up with, all in the name of money, fame, and entertainment, is beyond remarkable. It is insane, as "normal" as people treat it.

Long before them, and they still exist, were religious groups who engaged in terribly painful flagellation to test or prove their faith in God. Even *halachah*, on occasion, expects us to bite the bullet make great personal sacrifices to get the job done. Witness the deaths of Rebi Akiva and the rest of the Ten Martyrs who suffered terribly to protect Torah and the Jewish people.

The point is that it is amazing how much pain people are willing to undergo when the reason for doing so matters more to them than the reason for not doing so. Often too much, putting their futures on the line for things that do not matter as much as they think they do, or society has convinced them of.

The even deeper point is that this is a power that can be used for dealing with unavoidable pain. Obviously choosing pain makes it more meaningful, especially if there is a chance you can avoid much of it, or the worst part of it. But like with every difficult thing in life, a lot of extra pain comes from resisting it…from resenting it…from trying to escape it. Yes, will plays a role in the healing process, but not always the way people think.

The great Rebi Akiva suffered in many ways throughout his long life, but none as painful and as difficult as the last one.

> When they took Rebi Akiva out to be executed, it was the time for saying the *Shema*. They combed his flesh with iron combs while he accepted upon himself the yoke of the kingdom of Heaven…His soul left him as he was extending the word, *"Echad."* (*Brochos* 61b)

What a gruesome death. What a terribly painful way

to go. And yet when his students questioned his settled devotion to God at such an unsettling moment, he answered:

> "All of my life I have been bothered by the verse [in the *Shema* about loving God] *'with all of your soul'* (*Devarim* 6:5), which means, even if He *takes* your soul. I have asked myself, 'When will I be able to fulfill this?' Now that I have the opportunity, should I not fulfill it?"

Some say that at a certain point Rebi Akiva didn't even feel the pain anymore, perhaps because of the shock or even because of some miracle. True or not, he certainly felt the pain in the beginning because the Romans excelled at that. They just didn't realize who they were dealing with, someone who, unlike their other victims, not only accepted his situation but used it to his spiritual advantage.

My *Rosh Yeshivah* used to tell us that even the most difficult things in life often come down to a single decision that can be made in a moment. Once made, doing the difficult thing becomes just another part of life.

For example, it seems very hard to diet. People start and stop shortly after all the time. They think they have decided to diet, but they really haven't. They have decided to lose weight and that they want to be skinnier, but that doesn't mean they have also decided to eat less food. If they had, then going off their diet would become like eating *treif*—possibly tempting but never a possibility.

On the other hand, people who did make the decision to actually diet often talk about how easy it is to stay with it, even in the face of temptation. Violation of the diet feels like violation of the self, and kills the desire for illicit food.

The pain of denial even becomes pleasurable at some point because it acts as of a form of self-validation. It tells the person about themself, "I am in control of my will enough to do what I *want* to do, not what I *feel* like doing. I am in charge of me."

In fact, though a hero is anyone who saves the day for others, a *hero's* hero is someone who does it at personal cost. It is noble to care for others and help them out. It is even nobler when someone is willing to do it knowing that they will pay for it, whether this means financial layout, or jumping on a live grenade to save the lives of others knowing that it will kill them.

People talk about being heroic when they manage to smile as they frown inside because of terrible pain:

It was *Erev Simchas Torah* when the *Rosh Yeshivah* learned about the death of his son. But in a couple of hours, he knew that the joy of his entire *yeshivah* will depend upon his own joy of dancing with the Sefer Torah. So he willed himself to forget about his heartbreaking news for an entire day, not letting on to anyone about what happened to his family. Only after

Havdalah was made did the Rosh Yeshivah turn his attention to his personal tragedy and begin his mourning.

On another occasion, a certain rav entered the *Mir Bais Midrash* in Poland looking somewhat disheartened. Upon seeing this, the *Mashgiach Ruchani* told him, "I am sorry for your trouble. But though what you feel inside belongs to you, your face is in the *reshus harabim*—public domain. As such, you are obligated to be happy for others!"

Easier said than done. Sometimes inner pain is so intense it forces its way to the outside against our will. A face is called *panim*, a word that means *inside*, because it tends to reveal on the *outside* what a person feels on the *inside*. It's part of its job description, and it can take a great act of will to make it lie…a *heroic* act of will.

The funny thing about will is that it is so important for life and yet taken so for granted. It is such a powerful force in history, and yet so undervalued and underused. Yes, will ultimately must translate into physical action. But the level of commitment to carry out an act, and the Heavenly help a person receives to succeed at what they attempt, is very much tied to how much will the person summons.

At the end of the day, will is the only real game changer. Yet, so many people do not know how to generate it on their own, without some kind of outside stimulation. If they're not paying motivation speakers to inspire them, then they're using some form of entertainment to talk to to their inside and heat things up.

That's okay. It works, and great things have been accomplished that way. We all need some kind of carrot on a stick to make us run, especially when we'd rather not. Correction, when the *body* would rather not.

Because *we* do. Our soul, our essential will, lives to accomplish and do meaningful things. If it could, our soul would do them non-stop without taking any breaks. It's the body that the soul has to lug around through life that seeks out physical comfort and avoids anything that blocks it.

The reason an athlete can get their body on side is because they are after something the body can relate to and want. Victory. Fame. Money. The body naturally wants these things and will go to great extents to get them. Spiritual growth? A bigger portion in the World to Come? Doesn't talk to the body, and won't until it has concrete proof that it is its benefit to take the risk.

It's like trying to get investors for a new idea. Every new product can succeed or fail, and an investor will only risk their money once they are convinced that the odds of former are greater than those of the latter. The more sure they are, the more of their money they will be willing to risk.

Get up at 3:30 in the morning? Me? No way, no how! That is the middle of the night for me, prime sleep time. Or, at least it once was. Then one day I accidentally discovered the pleasure of *dovening* at *Neitz*

(Sunrise), which can get very early in the summer-time…and even *earlier* if you decide to come earlier to learn before *dovening*. All of a sudden, one day, I found myself *willingly* getting up each day at 3:30 in the morning, even when *Neitz* was later…even on the *chagim*. The pleasure of learning so early in the morning got my body into it as well, and there is something *heroic* about making such a sacrifice that talks to my body so that even *it* complains if we accidentally sleep in!

I recently heard a story about a Rosh Yeshivah who had lost his wife and ended up being late for the funeral. After he finally arrived, and everything that had to happen did, someone asked him where he had been.

"In my room," he answered.

"Can I ask what the *Rosh Yeshivah* was doing at that time?" the person pressed, curious about what had occupied the *Gadol's* time and made him late for such an important *mitzvah* and of someone so beloved.

"I was trying the find the *good* in what had happened," was all he said.

Good? What *good* could there have possibly been in the loss of a wife of so many years and such a righteous woman? Who even says that there has to be?

Nachum *Ish Gamzu* for one. He was famous for saying "*Gam zu l'tovah*—This too is for the good" in the face of adversity, including his own:

Nachum *Ish Gamzu* was blind in both eyes, both arms and legs were amputated, and his entire body was covered in boils. He lay in a dilapidated house, and the legs of his bed were placed in buckets of water so that ants should not climb onto him since he was unable to keep them off in any other way. Once his students wanted to remove his bed from the house and afterward remove his other vessels [afraid the house was about to collapse]. He told them: "My sons, remove the vessels first, and afterward remove my bed. I can guarantee you that as long as I am in the house it will not fall."

They removed the vessels and afterward they removed his bed, and immediately the house collapsed. His students said to him: "Rebi, since you are clearly a completely righteous person, as we have just seen that as long as you were in your house it did not fall, why has this suffering happened to you?"

He answered them: "I brought it upon myself. I was traveling along the road to my father-in-law's house, and my load was divided between three donkeys, one of food, one of drink, and one of delicacies. A poor person came and stood before me in the road and said, 'Rebi, feed me.' I told him: 'Wait until I unload the donkey, after which I will give you something to eat.' But I had not managed to unload the donkey before he died. [Distraught that my short delay had caused his death,] I fell upon his face and said: 'May my eyes which had no compassion on your eyes be blinded! May my hands which had no compassion on your hands be amputated! May my legs which had no compassion on your legs be amputated!' My mind did not rest until I said: 'May my whole body be covered in boils!'"

His students said to him: "Even so, how bad it is for us that we have seen you in this state!"

He told them: "How bad it would be for me if you had not seen me in this state!" (*Ta'anis* 21a)

How many people confronted by a similarly terrible life situation would look for the good in it, let alone find any? If anything, they have to fight against seeing only bad in adversity, especially extreme adversity. There have been a lot of people walking around through history who have been angry at God for what they have suffered. The *yetzer hara* has made *sure* of that.

It's only natural to expect good in life and be upset when you get bad instead. *Natural*, but not *logical*.

Take health for example. As one doctor told a complaining patient, "Don't ask me why you're sick. Ask me why you're not sick more often, or worse! When you consider the billions of things that could go wrong, *should* go wrong with our bodies, it's amazing that whatever does work does work as well as it does, and for so many years!"

The trouble with something that works consistently is that you come to expect it, as if it is obligated to. We start to treat it like a right, which means that when it is taken away from us we feel wronged…and complain…and then fight to get back what we have come to believe is rightfully ours.

One of the Ten Commandments is a *mitzvah* to honor one's parents. What is the basis of this *mitzvah*, asked the *Chinuch*[1] and answers, *hakaras hatov*, the *mitzvah* to acknowledge the good someone has done for you. Honoring one's parents is a way of saying, "Thank you for bringing me into this world and giving me the opportunity of life."

But how many children feel this way about life or their parents? How many children who accept and perform this *mitzvah* do it because it is a *mitzvah*, like any other, or because they really feel *hakaras hatov* to their parents for life? Ironically, the more people have to grow up with, the more they seem to accept as if it is rightfully theirs, and not requiring any show of appreciation.

What they don't realize is that such an attitude only leads to disappointment, and then pain. A story from the *Gemora* makes this point. It is about Marta *bas* Baysos, a

---

[1] The *Sefer HaChinuch,* written in 13th-century Spain by an anonymous "Levi of Barcelona" systematically discusses the 613 Commandments.

wealthy Jewish woman who lived during the siege of Jerusalem by the Romans. Jewish rebels had destroyed reserves of food, and it wasn't long before even the pampered among those living in the Walled City had become desperate and had to go in search of their own food.

According to one opinion in the *Gemora*, Marta had been walking barefoot through the streets looking for food when she stepped on something that, though it might disgust anyone, it would not kill them.[2] But for Marta, it so overwhelmed her that she actually died from it, prompting Rabban Yochanan *ben* Zakkai to say concerning her: *"The tender and delicate woman among you who would not adventure to set the sole of her foot upon the ground."*[3]

Even our immune systems work in a similar way. Doctors develop an immunity to many sicknesses because they remain constantly exposed to them, forcing their immune systems to constantly battle them. This strengthens their immune system.

The rest of us who avoid every sickness like the plague run the risk of developing vulnerabilities to them, should we be exposed to them at some point. We slowly introduce children to different foods so that their digestive systems can adjust to them.

The bottom line? Entitlement has its place in life, but

---

[2] *Gittin* 56a.
[3] *Devarim* 28:56.

too great a sense of *magia lee*[4] undermines a person's ability to deal with the less friendly parts of life. Remember? When the going gets *tough*, the *tough* get going. Adversity and the pain it can bring is not an accidental part of life, but part-and-parcel with why we're here in the first place, a *huge* discussion of its own.

We've had some of that discussion in bits and pieces in previous chapters. But there is something else to talk about before because closing out a book on the profound and meaningful purpose of pain in life.

------

[4] Hebrew for, "it's coming to me."

nine

ouldn't we like to know? What's God thinking, and why? It would be so helpful to know this, even with Torah to guide us, because history is always changing and so much happens that we just don't understand.

It's also the point of Creation. Since the beginning, God has had something in mind that He has been revealing to us ever since we first walked the earth. A billion things may be going on at the same time, but all of them are a bite of information to help us figure out what God is thinking.

Sounds simple? It's actually very *kabbalistic*.

Let's say you're a Physics professor who understands Quantum Physics like the back of your hand. Then, one day, a colleague with zero background in the topic asks you for a clear and succinct explanation of what you teach. Where do you *begin*? *How* do you begin? How will you translate something so theoretical and extremely abstract into simple, non-frustrating everyday terms?

Not easy, very unlikely, and perhaps even *impossible*. And all of *that* exists on the side of *Yaish*. It may be theoretical and abstract, but it is still part of the world of *Yaish*, the physical world that it describes and from where it has been taken. How much more impossible is it to extract and explain knowledge from the realm of *Ayin*.

Ayin means *nothing*, but *kabbalistically*, it is the most something anything can be. What we call *reality* is really a much lesser watered down version of it, because nothing is more real than God. The fact that God seems so abstract or missing from a person's reality is their shortcoming, not His. Closing your eyes does not make the world go away, just your ability to see it.

Kabbalah is full of ironies, and this is the biggest of all. How can *something* so *something* be so *nothing*? That's easy. It just has to be super spiritual compared to something very physical. The light of God on the level of *Keser* is so spiritual and unfiltered compared to the light of God that permeates our physical existence that it is, to us, as if it doesn't exist.

But as God told Moshe *Rabbeinu* who wanted a peek at such a high level of light:

You will not be able to see My face, for no man can

That goes against the purpose of Creation. We're not here to have a momentary relationship with God and then move on to the next world. We're here to become aware of God, increase our awareness of Him and eventually develop a personal and close relationship with God, as much as humanly possible.

It's like electricity. At its source, electricity is too powerful for everyday human use. So, we step it down and weaken it until we can use it without blowing anything up. But it would never make it to our communities if it wasn't strong at its source because it gets weaker as it travels through electrical cables over long distances.

But that's electricity. It's physical. We're talking about taking *infinite* and completely spiritual light and making it less infinite spiritual light so something physical can exist and even relate to it…so we can know what God is thinking.

In this respect, life is like a painting. When a master paints, every brush stroke conveys a message, what the artist was thinking when he painted it. It can be a conscious thought or an unconscious one, but it might as well be an envelope waiting to be opened by the person trying to decipher their work, with a message inside that says, "This is what I was thinking when I painted this."

The translation of God's abstract thought into ideas that we can grasp is called *Chochmah*—Wisdom. *In the se-*

firos, Chochmah is the next level down after *Keser* (*Ayin*) because that is what it does, it transforms the light of *Ayin* into the light of *Yaish...yaish m'ayin*—something from nothing.

Wisdom is different from knowledge. Knowledge—*dayah*—is just fact without understanding, and will have no impact on the person who knows it. The moment knowledge impacts a person's level of understanding and *improves* their spiritual quality of life, it becomes *Chochmah,* and a revelation of Divine thought.

Now, this is something that happens everyday and all the time, sometimes in major ways, sometimes in small ways. Therefore, people take it for granted and tend not to appreciate the power of it, *unless something happens to make them*.

Something, like *suffering*.

It's not the ideal way, at least that is what we have been told and how it seems to us. But everything God does, and He does *everything*, is always ideal, perfect. He can never do anything less than the perfect thing, no matter how *imperfect* His actions seem to us. Perfection can only breed perfection.

But *ideal* and *less than ideal* are realities for us free will beings so that our choices in life can have real consequences. The ideal way to gain *Chochmah* is by learning Torah and performing *mitzvos*. Torah is a personal note from God, and *mitzvos* are expressions of His expectations. Both, when approached this way, are the most *direct* and *accurate* ways for knowing what's on God's mind.

But when they're not approached this way, which makes Torah just another area of religious study, and *mitzvos* just ways to stay in step with society, we learn nothing about God's thinking. And since the goal of Creation is to facilitate this, a third means was created to help with that, and we call it *tza'ar*—pain.[1]

Pain is *physical*, even *emotional* pain. It affects our brains, which affects our bodies. Sad or depressed people can't press a part of their body and feel pain as if it was a bruise, but their bodies slow down and have difficulty doing things as if their pain is physical.

Although we know quite well that we can psychologically manage pain, it is so much harder than popping a pill that will quickly mask it, or to do something distracting that will temporarily take our minds off of our pain. Pain is a medical issue to be dealt with medically. If pain teaches us anything, it is to try and avoid when possible the thing that led to it in the first place.

This makes pain and suffering an unfortunate and incidental part of life. We treat it like a flaw, a handicap that we were born with because of some error in our genetic code. Had *we* made man, we would have most certainly fixed that problem and done away with pain altogether, as geneticists have been trying to do for some time, with limited success.

---

[1] *Drushei Olam HaTohu, Chelek* 2, *Drush* 4, *Anaf* 19, *Siman* 6.

But that is not the way God sees pain. Pain is *profound*. Yes, it brings out the worst in some people, and maybe that is what it was meant to do for them, reveal their spiritual weaknesses. People are good at pretending to be stronger than they are until they're proven otherwise by pain.

But pain also brings out the best in many others. What heroic act would be considered complete if it didn't also come at the cost of some personal pain? We measure greatness by a person's level of will to do good, and nothing measures strength of will better than resistance to pain for a higher cause. This impresses us and, if the hero happens to die in the process, we will make a point of eulogizing them with it.

All true and deeply meaningful. But even more profound is the story and message of *Sefer Iyov*. Stepping back and appreciating the work for what it is, it is really quite amazing how many important ideas, many *kabbalistic*, are learned as a result of one righteous person's suffering.

On the surface of it, the story of Iyov is of a man who happened to be in the wrong place at the wrong time. His idyllic life was destroyed seemingly because of a bet between God and the *Satan*, that Iyov would stay his righteous course despite all of his sudden and seemingly illogical suffering.

Iyov *does*, until he *doesn't*.

It is not clear whether Iyov actually questioned God, or just began to have doubts in his heart about Divine justice. Either way, it led to a deep and philosophical discussion meant to widen the perspective on life of *everyone*, not only Iyov, and especially those who suffer. The bottom line: personal suffering is not only personal, but part-and-parcel of the overall plan for Creation, which no one but God understands.

It is also the basis of a *nisayon*, a Divinely-engineered test which God seems to be big on. Witness the *Avos* and all of their tests, and all the trials and tribulations of countless Jewish communities over the ages. Sometimes it seems that being Jewish means living from test to test.

But such tests are never to prove to *God* who we are and what we are capable of, because He already knows that before we do. Each test is carefully designed to answer the question, "Who are you really?" but not for God. It's for us, because we rarely do enough soul searching to find that out.

And a *nisayon* is not a test if it does not challenge us. A challenge is only a challenge when it makes life difficult, and a *difficult* life is a *painful* one. The more difficult life is, the more painful it will be, and the more it will reveal about the person…the better they will know themself.

It sounds kind of silly. How can we live with ourselves for so many years, think we know ourselves and yet, not know our true selves much at all? But the answer to that question stares us in the face everyday that we see our reflection, and see a *body*, not a *soul*.

I remember once as a teenager I was crossing the

road and passed an elderly person struggling with some packages. Without giving it a second thought, I ran to help them with their bags across the road, and only once I felt they were safely across did I return the packages and went my way.

They, of course, thanked me profusely, which of course made me feel good. But what made me feel even better was how I had run to help without thinking about it, like it was the most natural thing to do. I could have pretended to not have noticed the person in distress and kept going on my way, as others seemed to be doing.

What surprised me the most when I considered how upbeat I felt from such a simple act of kindness was how surprised I was by what I did, and how reassured it made me feel. It was like some kind of confirmation to me that I was, in essence, a good person. I realized then and there how much a stranger I was to myself, though until that time I wouldn't have known it.

The second major time this happened to me it was many years later, far more dramatic, and changed my life *forever.* The details are not that important, but the result was, which was to make me investigate my life until that time, to find out who I *really* was inside.

My investigation took about a year, and meant collecting as many pictures of me over the years, and interviewing as many people I could who knew me growing up. It was a lot of fun and very instructional because I was told things about myself over the years that I never paid much attention to, if at all.

I also spent time trying to remember as much as I could as far back as I could, and that alone was quite an experience. It is really quite amazing how easy it is to forget things from your past if they weren't traumatic, and how possible it is to re-access them if you make a mental effort to do so.

Though most details weren't significant on their own, they were nevertheless important pieces of all the overall puzzle of who I was to that point in my life that was forming before my very eyes, or rather, my *mental* eye. And even if I didn't have the whole picture, I was starting to feel a wonderful feeling of *shlaimus*—personal completion—I had only felt on occasion and only for brief moments in the past.

Obviously there were many details I left out on my journey of self-discovery, either because I had to move or they just weren't available to me anymore. But it didn't matter, because at some point I really felt as if I had a better idea of who I was in essence, at least enough of a base to build upon as I learned more about life and me in the future.

Where all of this eventually had the greatest impact was in my relationship with God, especially during *tefillah*. It is one thing to stand before God. It is something very different to stand before God as *you*. Once you do, you want to do it even more, which forces a person to become more them, and that is what I work on everyday, and especially on *Yom Kippur*.

Because *Yom Kippur* is a special day. And though everyone already knows that, too few people know it in the way mentioned earlier.[2] They know it as a serious day, a day of fasting, a day of long prayers…a day that a Jew has to put up with and go along with because, well, that's what Jews do.

And maybe that is all that God expects from many of us. Every army has its soldiers whose job it is not to question commands or innovate an attack, but to simply follow orders and carry out the strategies of higher-ups. That is exactly what a person does who fulfills all the *halachos* of *Yom Kippur* even though they gain no additional knowledge about God, themself, and their relationship.

But should that not be enough for a person, and if they feel that *Yom Kippur* has more to offer them if they offer more to *Yom Kippur*, then they should move to Plan B:

> I used to feel a certain dread once *Rosh Chodesh Elul* began. The blowing of the *shofar* together with the addition of the prayer *L'Dovid* meant that the summer was officially over, and it was time to get more serious about life. Soon we would begin *Selichos*, adding even more prayer and time to the regular *tefillah*. Rosh Hashanah, of course, would follow with

---

[2] See Chapter 6.

its many hours spent in *shul*. That would lead to eight more days of seriousness that would culminate in the fast and prayer-filled day of *Yom Kippur.* Whatever my *soul* felt about all of that was drowned out by the kicking, screaming, and resistance of my body. All I could do was what was expected of me, and look forward to when it would all be over again. But with age comes maturity, and even a little wisdom. It was a gradual process over many years, but eventually I turned *Yom Kippur* from being only God's day into my day, and then eventually into *our* day. All that time spent in prayer and trying to connect to God became a special time for me to connect to myself as well. As I mentally fought to feel the Presence of God in my life, as if I was literally standing right before Him, I had to cut through all the layers of self-percep-tion I had built up over the years. The more I did this, the more I felt "me," and the better I felt about it. More importantly, I felt so much closer to God...ac-tually feeling the Presence of God. It is such an awe-some and exhilarating feeling, like a treasure found at the end of a long and difficult search that makes the journey worth it in the end. Now, many years later, when *Rosh Chodesh Elul* begins I feel *no* dread, only joy. For me, now, it means that my journey to my long-lost "friend" has begun, and I become excited with anticipation of actually being in His Presence once again.

That person gets it. And because they do, their quality of life will be very high. They'll be better-equipped to deal with adversity, and able to help others with theirs. Beyond that, they will become someone God can work with, and talk to, in one way or another. They'll have a much better understanding of what is on God's mind.

ten

Laughter is the best medicine, *or so the expression goes.* And though it can't always be the best medicine at every time, it certainly is a good one at the right time.

It does have a medicinal effect:

It's true: laughter is strong medicine. It draws people together in ways that trigger healthy physical and emotional changes in the body. Laughter strengthens your immune system, boosts mood, diminishes pain, and protects you from the damaging effects of stress. Nothing works faster or more dependably to bring your mind and body back into balance than a good laugh. Humor lightens your burdens, inspires hope, connects you to others, and keeps you grounded, focused, and alert. It also helps you release anger and forgive sooner. With so much power to heal and renew, the ability to laugh easily and frequently is a tremendous resource for surmounting problems, enhancing your relationships, and supporting both physical and emotional health. Best of all, this priceless medicine is fun, free, and easy to use. As children, we used to laugh hundreds of times a day, but as adults, life tends to be more serious and laughter more infrequent. But by seeking out more opportunities for humor and laughter, you can improve your emotional health, strengthen your relationships, find greater happiness—and even add years to your life.[1]

In other words, laughter is the opposite of pain. Everything pain causes, laughter has the opposite effect. We don't pay comedians just to make us laugh for entertainment's sake. Like motivational speakers, comedians provide something simple we all desperately need but have difficulty getting on our own.

But not all laughter. When laughter comes at the cost of something else important, like self-dignity, it loses a lot of its positive effect. People may find rude and coarse hu-

---

[1] Laughter may even help you to live longer. A study in Norway found that people with a strong sense of humor outlived those who don't laugh as much. The difference was particularly notable for those battling cancer (https://www.helpguide.org/mental-health/wellbeing/laughter-is-the-best-medicine).

mor funny but it is a cheap and undignified substitute for the real thing. As the *Zohar* says, what comes out of a person's mouth reveals their true nature.[2]

What is *real* humor? There are different sources of humor, but one of the greatest and most profound comes from something we call irony:

> Irony, in its broadest sense, is the juxtaposition of what on the surface *appears* to be the case and what is *actually* the case or to be expected.

When something is ironically *bad*, it hurts even more. Not only did you get a flat tire, but you got it the one time it happened to hail and you forgot to charge your phone so you could call for help. It is ironic that all three things happened at the same time, but not funny.

When something is ironically *good*, it can make a person laugh:

> *Avraham fell on his face and laughed, and he said to himself, "Will [a child] be born to one who is a hundred years old, and will Sarah, who is ninety years old, give birth?" (Bereishis 17:7)*

> *Sarah laughed to herself, saying, "After I have become worn out, will I have smooth flesh? And also,*

---

[2] *Zohar, Balak* 193b.

my master is old." (*Bereishis* 18:12)

In the first scenario, the special situation makes the person feel very *unspecial*. If they don't believe in God then they feel very unlucky, as if they're having a bad day. If they do believe in God, then they feel that He is out to get them, which hurts even more.

In the second scenario, the special result makes the person feel special, in a good way. If they don't believe in Divine Providence then they will attribute their unexpected success to good luck which, even though they believe it is random, still makes them special.

If the person *does* believe that God is behind their success, something they notice even more now because of the unexpected circumstances that led to it, they will feel blessed. They will feel that God is favoring them, which will definitely make them feel better about themself. For a believer, success is so much sweeter when it seems like a gift from God:

> *Sarah said, "God has made laughter for me; whoever hears will laugh about me…Who would have said to Avraham that Sarah would nurse children, for I have borne a son to his old age!"* (*Bereishis* 21:6-7)

It says, regarding the final redemption:

A song of ascents. When God returns the returnees to Tzion, we will be like dreamers. Then our mouths will be filled with laughter and our tongues with songs of praise. Then they will say among the nations, "God has done great things with these." (Tehillim 12:1-2)

Why *laughter*? Because the final redemption will be an ultimate act of irony. After all, the world does not look at the Jewish people in any special way, and if anything, just the opposite. Anti-Semitism once again is increasingly quickly around the world, endangering Jews everywhere they live.

Even many Jews themselves have drifted towards the gentile point of view about their own people. Just imagine how they're going to react when God finally reveals Himself to the world and makes it clear that the Torah was, is, and will always be real. Tremendous regret will be the least of their problems.

But again, why *laughter*? Joy, *yes*. Exuberance, *yes*. Gratefulness, *unquestionably*. But what does laughter have to do with any of this?

Because at this stage of history it is difficult to be upbeat all the time, even for generally upbeat people. It is even easy for people to be sad and become depressed. Despite all the sources of pleasure and distraction that we have today, the rate of depression in all societies is very high. It's a world that can easily cause pain.

And it needs to be. From the time the first man was created until the time *Moshiach* will finally bring all evil to its eternal end, all of history will have been about man's use of free will. People go through much of their lives making choices as automatically as they do breathe, and almost just as unconsciously.

But not God. No human choice is too big or too small for Him not to take notice of it. And aside from taking note of each one and recording it for a person's day of judgment, God also uses them to determine who will be the good guys in history and who will be the bad ones. A choice today determines where God will plug you in tomorrow.

For choice to have any meaning it has to have consequence. There has to be a good consequence and a bad one, which means there has to be good and there has to be evil. There also has to be agents of good, like the *yetzer tov*, a person's inclination to do good which is the soul drive, and agents of evil, such as a *yetzer hara*, and bad angels like the *Satan*.

Pain can be the result of evil or good. When pain is caused through the abuse of others, it is evil. When it is a warning signal from the body to stop doing something harmful, it is good. When it's self-inflicted for no Godly reason, it is evil. When it is the result of trying to do what God wants, it is heroic.

There is a lot of pain in the world, and there has been since the beginning. Some of it is for good reasons, and a lot of it is because of evil. Either way, pain has been persistent, and we spend a lot of time and money trying to prevent it or at least manage it.

It has had a direct impact on people's faith in God. After all, what kind of God makes a world in which so many people can suffer so much and for so long? So they make the illogical (but convenient) assumption that God didn't make the world and instead focus on ways to limit the amount of pain man has to put up with.

They should have had a good laugh instead. It would have given them a taste of the better life. Having a good laugh is like being on an airplane during a terrible storm that is rocking the plane and rising up above the clouds where it is sunny and peaceful. The storm may be there when you go back down again, but at least for a moment you were able to feel good, safe, and have peace of mind.

Granted that a good laugh rarely has enough power to fix a damaged reality. No one is saying that it is supposed to. On the contrary, according to the *Gemora*, any pain we suffer is under contract to last as long as it does:

> Zunin asked Rebi Akiva, "We both know that idols have no power, so how is it that sometimes their worshippers come to them crippled and walk away healed?"
>
> He answered with a parable. "There was once a very honest person in a town whom people trusted, left their precious belongings in his safekeeping,

even without witnesses. One man however refused to rely on the man's honesty and insisted upon witnesses being on hand when he left something. On one occasion however he left something with the man but forgot to bring witnesses. The guardian's wife suggested that they deny ever receiving the deposit. 'Because this fool acts improperly,' he said, 'we should abandon our faithfulness?' Likewise," Rebi Akiva said, "when suffering is sent from Heaven to afflict a person, it is bound by strict contract when to come and leave, and at precisely which hour to stop, and in response to which healer and medicine it must be cured. If at the appointed time to leave the sufferer visits an idol's temple the illness [at first] says, 'It is only right that we do not leave,' but then concludes, 'Because this fool has acted improperly we should abandon our faithfulness to the oath we took?'" (*Avodah Zarah* 55a)

Instead, a good, clean laugh is like taking a painkiller. A painkiller does not solve the problem of the source of pain. It just prevents the nervous system from transmitting the feeling of pain:

When we are in pain or injured, a protein called COX2 releases chemicals called prostaglandins. These chemicals send a signal to your brain, telling you you're in pain. Painkillers like aspirin, ibuprofen and paracetamol bind to COX2 , preventing it from producing any more prostaglandins. This reduces pain. (5medicine-makers_web_flyer_190x240-1.pdf)

Isn't that cheating? If God is the one inflicting the pain, aren't we just asking for more trouble by deflecting it?

Yes, *sometimes*. But pain is a motivator, and God can use it to motivate a person to do many things. Maybe the person is being made to suffer so they will have to go to a doctor, get a prescription, fill it, take it, and who knows what else. God knows what He wants from a person, what they need to do, and exactly how to get them to do it.

And what about all the other people involved? They'll also be affected as they are meant to be affected, whether they're a relative, employer, doctor, pharmacist, or whoever we impact with our life's situations. It's all exquisitely Divinely orchestrated because, when you're God, you can do the seemingly incredible or impossible without making any errors. We don't believe in coincidences or accidents, even if we call them that.

Even tickling is interesting. Why should a good tickle cause laughter? That's like saying, why does a little alcohol make you feel better about life even if life is not better? It is a gift from the Creator that such superficial stimulation should be able to help us cope with life so we can use our time to our best advantage. Used wisely, they can help. Abused, they can destroy.

More *kabbalistically*, pain and laughter are really

two opposite forces built into and run Creation. Pain is a function of *tzimtzum*, the constriction of God's light which is a function of the light of *Gevurah*. In the right amount it is the basis of discipline and judgment (Yitzchak), but in extreme amounts it is the basis of evil (Eisav).

Which is ironic since laughter is a function of *Chesed*, kindness, the trait of Avraham *Avinu*. It is a *chesed* that we can laugh and a *chesed* when we make others laugh because of all the positive effects of doing so. That's why making people laugh in a honest way usually results in another important and elusive trait, *chayn*.

It was *chayn* that Noach found in the eyes of God that saved him from the Flood, and *chayn* that made Yosef *HaTzaddik* so successful against the odds. Children are known for *chayn* which is not surprising. We learned earlier that they are also big on humor.

It is clear from Torah that *chayn* can be superficial or profound. When translated as charm or external beauty, it is not very profound at all. But when *chayn* is the light of a person's soul exuding to the outside world for people to see and experience, the result of self-sacrifice for a noble cause, then it is the profoundest reality of all.

This is why undignified humor and humor that makes others feel bad about themselves does not cause the comic to give off *chayn*. They might be funny, but not *chaynadik*. They might entertain, but they won't have optimal healing effect.

Another underrated aspect of laughter is sarcasm. It's

trickier than regular humor because it is much easier to get it wrong than a simple joke that might flop, especially since sarcasm tends to be based upon reality.

For example, when the Jewish people got to the Red Sea, they found themselves stuck between a hard rock and a wall. Actually, between a killer sea and a killer army, the Egyptians had chased after them and pinned them down by the sea. But it led (at least in my opinion) to one of the greatest sarcastic lines of all time:

> *They said to Moshe, "Is it because there are no graves in Egypt that you have taken us to die in the desert?" (Shemos* 14:11)

Picture the scene. Millions of Jews, men, women, children, elderly, healthy, infirmed, fresh out of slavery thinking they had seen the last of their Egyptian taskmasters. Then, quite suddenly and terrifyingly, they find themselves with a deadly sea on one side and a ruthless army on the other side. Who wouldn't panic in such a situation?

Those who could speak to Moshe didn't say to him, "Moshe, now what?" or, "How can we cross the sea…or defend ourselves against the Egyptian army?" They didn't ask him, "Okay, where is God now when we need Him the most?"

No, instead they said to Moshe, "Hey Moshe! What, there weren't enough places back in Egypt to bury us so you took us out into the desert where there's plenty of room to bury us here?" Pure sarcasm.

Yes, sarcasm bites. But in it is also one of the most important ingredients for surviving any crisis: hope. Cynicism, what Amalek promotes, says that there is no hope. Sarcasm says that the situation *should* be, *could* be better than it is, *so why isn't it?* The mocking of the situation is actually part of an effort to make it better, if not this time, then maybe in the future.

Because nothing keeps a cause going longer than the hope that success is still possible, that it can get better somehow, some way. And nothing shuts down a person faster than the killing of any hope they might have hung on to, the main thing Jewish enemies have worked on doing most.

And laughter? It's an injection of hope. It may not talk about the hope or describe it in any tangible way. But the positiveness that laughter causes and the good feeling it leaves a person feeling somehow also translates into some kind of feeling of hope that life is good, or that it can be better.

The *Gemora* talks about how a certain rabbi, while talking to Eliyahu *HaNavi* in a marketplace, wanted to know who was guaranteed a portion the World to Come. Eliyahu pointed out someone who, to the rabbi, did not look the part at all. "*He's* guaranteed a portion in the World to Come?" the rabbi asked incredulously. "*Why?*"

"Because," Eliyahu answered him, "he makes people laugh."

You can be sure that not every standup comedian is guaranteed a portion in the World to Come, if they're going there at all, especially if they were foul-mouthed or immodest. But a handful might be just because of the clean and kind way they lifted people spirits and gave them perspective and hope, if only for a few joyous moments.

It is also more than interesting that the Jewish holiday that seems the least holiday is actually the most holy, especially since it involves laughter. The *Midrash* says that all the Jewish holidays will eventually be annulled because the light they allowed temporary access to during our period of history will be fully accessible in the next one.[3]

However, they will not all disappear at once. *Chanukah*, which allows access to the light of the Messianic Era will be the first to stop being a holiday in Yemos *HaMoshiach* when everyday will be *Chanukah. Rosh Hashanah, Pesach, Shavuos, Succos, and Shemini Atzeres,* are lights from the next period after that of *Techiyas HaMeisim*, the Resurrection of the Dead, so they will no longer be necessary as holidays at that time.

At 6,000, this world will end and the World to Come will begin in stages as Creation becomes increasingly holier. The first stage, the seventh millennium, is called *Olam HaNeshamos*, the *World of the Souls*, and is called "the day that is completely *Shabbos.*" This means that everyday will radiate the light of *Shabbos*, not just the seventh day of

---

[3] *Yalkut Shimoni, Mishlei, Remez* 940.

week, so *Shabbos* will stop being a special day in that time.

At 7,000, the world will reach the level of the light of *Yom Kippur*, making the eighth millennium *"the day that is completely Yom Kippur."* We won't need to pray all day or fast then, because we only need things like that during this phase of history while still in our bodies so we can access that light. During the eighth millennium, we'll just bask in it with eternal pleasure.

At that time, the only holiday left, whatever that will mean at that difficult-to-fathom stage of the World to Come, will be *Purim*. The light of *Purim* won't be a daily occurrence until the *ninth* millennium, from 8,000 onward, which corresponds to the second highest *sefirah* of *Chochmah*.

Talk about counterintuitive.[4] What often ends up be-

---

[4] It says in *Megillas Esther*, *"on the day that the enemies of the Jews looked forward to ruling over them, it was reversed—nahafoch hu…"* (*Esther* 9:1). *Nahafoch hu* can be read *Nun-hafuch*—upside-down *Nun*, or in this case, the righting of the upside-down *Nun*. The *Gemora* recounts this story: Rebi Yehoshua's son became weak and his soul left him. When he recovered, his father asked him, "What did you see?" He answered him, "An upside-down world! [There], whoever is esteemed here, was down, and those who are down [here] were esteemed." He told him, "My son, you saw a clear world!" (*Pesachim* 50a). In other words, *Purim* is the juxtaposition of the next world in our world, which looks upside down to us because we live upside down to it. As Rebi Yehoshua told his son, "We're the one's walking on the ceiling," so-to-speak. That irony is the source of the humor to those who understand and relate to this truth.

ing the least holy Jewish holiday of the year down here at this stage of history is actually the result of a light that is holier than even the light of *Yom Kippur*. As they say, *Yom KiPurim*—a day *like Purim*. It just goes to show how much of an impact spiritual environment has on the nature of someone or something.

It is any wonder then that we tend to associate a good sense of *good* humor with cleverness?

Have you ever seen a hippopotamus hiding in a tree? That's how good they are at it.

It is absurd to think that something so big as a hippo could climb a tree let alone hide in one. The obvious answer of the average brain would be, "No, and it is silly to even ask such a question."

So when the punchline ignores all of that and says that you can't see such a thing, but not because it is physically impossible, but because hippos are so good at doing it, you are surprised, duped, but in a funny kind of way. It is the absurd casually and comfortably made even more absurd, and *that's* funny.

Sometimes jokes are just the result of people sitting around making up material for some comedy act. But the funniest things in life are usually the result of someone seeing or learning something insightful that others may not see, or think of in that way. Someone with a certain perspective found the irony or absurdity in something the rest of us just take for granted as normal, and then shared their vision with us through a joke.

We could spend some time at this point sharing jokes and puns and gain important insights and perhaps, share a few laughs. One of my favorites?

Once there four rabbis, friends and colleagues who on occasion would take a walk together. They would use this time to discuss issues and share ideas, but invariably their discussions would always come down to a single point over which they would argue, always the same three against the same one.

On one particular outing it happened again, but with a difference. A specific issue was raised that ended up becoming an argument with the three rabbis taking exception with the fourth. This time, however, the lone dissenter was not going to take defeat easily.

"I'm tired," he said warily, "of always being the odd man out, especially *this* time when I am sure that I am *right*!"

"Well," said one of the other three rabbis, "the Torah does say that in cases such as this that the majority rules. So," he finished with a grin, "unless you have another three opinions to support yours, our majority opinion rules again!"

But this time the lone rabbi was not deterred. He had anticipated such a response and had already planned his countermove. He was going to do something radical because, from where he stood, he felt he had nothing to lose.

"What if," he said slyly, "*Heaven* agrees with me?"

The three rabbis looked at each other quizzically. "And just how do you intend to prove that?" one of them asked.

"With a Divine sign!" he said provocatively.

"*A Divine sign?*" another questioned. "Really? And just *how* do you intend to do that?"

"Like this!" he answered, turning his eyes Heavenward and saying, "Dear God, please forgive me this bold request, which I make in fear and in trepidation. But, as You know, whenever my colleagues and I get into an argument it is always the three of them against me. In the past I have accepted that maybe I was wrong, and kept my peace. This time, however, I know I am right but am incapable of convincing my colleagues. Therefore I ask You, not for *my* sake, but for the sake of Your eternal truth, to provide some sign that clearly proves to my fellow rabbis that I have the correct opinion in this particular matter."

Having concluded his request, he became silent and waited. The other three rabbis, incredulous, felt obligated to wait a few moments before mocking his attempt to drag Heaven into their disagreement. But before they could, a cloud suddenly appeared out of nowhere above them in the otherwise clear sky. As they looked at it in wonder, the cloud rumbled for several moments and then disappeared as fast and mysteriously as it had first appeared.

The four rabbis continued to stand in their places transfixed for several minutes. Even the rabbi who had requested the sign was completely surprised by the occurrence, until one of the other three rabbis finally said something.

"Unquestionably that mysterious cloud was Divine Providence, especially given the otherwise perfectly clear blue and the timing of the cloud's arrival and the rumbling sound it made. But," he added before the fourth rabbi could feel vindicated, "that was *all* it was, interesting...It does not conclusively prove that Heaven agrees with your opinion. And besides," he added for good measure while the other rabbis nodded in agreement, "the Torah has already told us that Heavenly signs no longer decide earthly matters."

"Maybe," the lone rabbi answered, "but I'm not leaving here today until it is clear that my opinion is Heaven's opinion too!"

Emboldened by their dissonance, the dissenting rabbi again turned his gaze towards Heaven and made a second impassioned plea: "Dear Almighty! Far be it from me to bother You for such trivial matters as a simple little argument. However, now my friends over here even doubt Your sign! So, if it is at all possible, please send one that indisputably shows them the truth of the matter . . ."

Before the other rabbis could protest against such a request, the cloud returned looking even more foreboding than the first time. It rumbled again, but this time lightning came down and actually hit the tree next to them, splitting it in two and leaving it smoldering.

All of them could neither move nor speak. They were all firm believers in Divine Providence, but none of them had ever experienced such a blatant example of it. Clearly it was a miracle, a *big* miracle.

Or was it? As the moments of silence ticked away, the *yetzer hara* had time to do its thing. Doubt began to creep into the minds of the three rabbis, and it wasn't long before one of them finally said, "Granted what we all just witnessed was completely out of the ordinary. But," he continued while looking for the agreement of others, "it doesn't prove that you are right about anything!"

"Yes," said one of the other two. "How do we know that the whole thing is not just Heaven's way of saying don't invoke Divine signs?"

"Are you kidding me?" the fourth rabbi asked, incredulous and frustrated. "After all that…and after putting myself on the line like that…you're going to write the whole thing off and maintain your positions?"

They looked at each other and, nodding, answered, "Well, *yes*."

He shook his head in disbelief and said, "Well, that's it for me. I've already done far more than I should have to make my point. If you're going to continue to be so stubborn, that's your business…"

But before he could finish his sentence, a very loud and awesome voice called out from above them, *"Heeee's RIGHT!"*

No one moved for what seemed like an eternity. It was clear where the voice had come from and this time, its message was indisputably clear: God sided with the single opinion.

But as they all considered what just happened and what it means, one of the three rabbis concluded and said, "Okay…fine…you've made your point. So now it's *three against two.*"

I won't know whether you laughed at this joke or not, or even if you find this kind of humor funny. I do know that if you read all of it, I distracted you from life for a few moments, and that allowed you to forget about whatever it is that might be bothering you.

At the very least, you might have felt a little better about life, if only for a few moments. But even a few moments of improved quality of life is a *chesed*, and that is what we were created to receive, and are encouraged to do for others.

Strength and beauty are her raiment, and she

laughs at the last day. (*Mishlei* 31:25)

laughs at the last day. (Mishlei 31:25)

Other Books

The Fabric of Reality

Fundamentals of Reincarnation

Reincarnation Clarified

All About Energy

What Goes Around

The God Experience, Part 1

What in Heaven

The God Experience, Part 2

The God Experience, Part 3

It's About Time

Need to Know

Perceptions, Volume 2

Once Revealed, Twice Concealed

The Art of *Chayn*

A Matter of Laugh or Death

Geulah b'Rachamim Program, 1

Geulah b'Rachamim Program, 2

Geulah b'Rachamim Program, 3

Point of Acceptance

See Ya

In Discussion: *Bereishis*

Reincarnation Again

A Separate Matter

In Discussion: *Shemos*

A Search for Self

A Search for Trust

In Discussion: *Bamidbar*

How It Might Play Out

In Discussion: *Vayikra*

Where Are My Emotions Now

In Discussion: *Devarim*

Oh, So Blind

Not So Bad?

Sha'ar HaPesukim (Translation)

The Fix

Preparing For Redemption

Mindfulness, Torah & Redemption

Moment of Moments

My *Zaidy's* Diary

My Writing, Your Book

Living Higher

Landing Higher

A Matter of Choice

Loose Ends

In Pursuit of Wisdom

What The Doctor Ordered

Estimated Time of Arrival

Tell Me More (Children's Book)

More About Me

Tell Me More Again (Children's Book)

What's Really Going On

Leshem, Volume 1 (Translation)

Leshem, Volume 2 (Translation)

Highest Knowledge Ever

Happiness Please

World of Lies

Half Full

Truth From Heaven

Vayechulu

Strategy For The End of Days

Leshem, Volume 3 (Translation)

Inspired
Haggadah Shel Pesach
Don't Panic
Leshem On The Parsha
Run Pain, Run

The books are available in Kindle, Paperback, PDF, or Hardcover formats as well. PDF books can be purchased in the Thirtysix.org online bookstore, and the other formats are available through Amazon.com. For additional information, write to:

pinchasw@thirtysix.org